"This book is an intimate and honest account of a cancer patient's journey, who happens to be an Oncology Nurse. It is inspirational, insightful, and authentic! As an Oncology Social Worker, I would recommend that my patients read Christine's story and experience how she learned to cope with cancer and live life to the fullest."

—Kathy Yeatman-Stock, MSW, LCSW, OSW-C
Licensed Oncology Clinical Social Worker
PVHMC Robert & Beverly Lewis Cancer Care Center

"Whether you are a Health care professional, or a lay person, you will find 'Both Sides of the Bedside' making you chuckle, cry and smile all the way to the end. It is easy to read and it gives you a great perspective as to what it means to care for people with cancer and then be a person with cancer fighting this disease. Great read!"

—Enza Esposito-Nguyen, RN, MSN, ANP-BC
Oncology Nurse Practitioner/Nurse Navigator

"Christine Magnus Moore has written a heartfelt book about her experiences as an oncology nurse and non-Hodgkin Cancer Survivor. We walk the path with her from the time of diagnosis through her cancer treatment and beyond. What is remarkable about this is that she did that sharing the events and her emotions, spirituality, insight and knowledge. She both mirrored what she and many others experience but did it in a way that is both affirming and educational. This book will be of tremendous value to anyone walking this path-be that the person with cancer or their family, friends or co-workers."

—Deborah K. Mayer, PhD, RN, AOCN, FAAN
Professor, School of Nursing
Director of Cancer Survivorship
UNC Lineberger Comprehensive Cancer Center
University of North Carolina, Chapel Hill, NC

"Christine has written an insightful look into the pain, fear, courage and hope of a young woman's journey as she battles the disease of cancer. This is an especially compelling read for those of us who have never had cancer nor cared for someone who has. Whether a health care worker, family member or friend I highly recommend this book - you will be blessed and impacted at the same time!"

—David E. Rice, Ph.D., Marriage and Family Therapist

Both Sides of the Bedside

BOTH SIDES OF THE BEDSIDE

From Oncology Nurse to Patient, an RN's Journey with Cancer

Christine Magnus Moore, RN, BSN

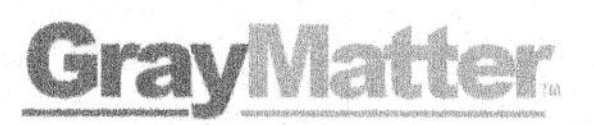

Gray Matter Imprints
Irvine, California

Both Sides of the Bedside:
From Oncology Nurse to Patient, an RN's Journey with Cancer

Printed in the United States of America

The content contained in this book is based on the author's experiences and is intended for informational and educational purposes only. It is not a medical instruction manual and is not to be used as a medical handbook. It does not replace obtaining medical treatment and advice. This book offers experiences and wisdom gained by the author, but the author is in no way suggesting medical advice or direction.
There are references to websites which are not under the control of the author or publisher. The author has no control over the nature and content on those sites. The inclusion of the links does not necessarily imply a recommendation or endorse the views expressed on them.

Book cover design by Corinne Gronnel
www.GraphicallyInspired.com

Book cover image Copyright Poznyakov, used under license from Shutterstock.com

Some proceeds from this book will be donated to cancer-related charities.

ISBN-13: 978-0986285356
ISBN-10: 0986285358
Library of Congress Control Number: 2015900515
Gray Matter Imprints, Irvine, CA

This book is dedicated to those who gave me the privilege of helping them during their trials, and for anyone who will allow me to help them as a result of my own.

To my mom who has loved me amidst all my foibles, fumbles and follies. Thank you for your incredible heart, a constant source of abundant love and caring. Thank you for being my biggest cheerleader!

To my dad who has always viewed the world through colorful glasses. Your wit, wisdom and courage inspire me deeply.

To the Lord above. Thank you for giving me incredible opportunities!

Contents

Author's Note:

Included in this book is a collection of patient and co-worker interactions which occurred over a twenty-year time-period. While all the stories in this book are true, I have maintained privacy and confidentiality by altering identifying characteristics, and sometimes circumstances, in patients and health care professionals. For those whose real names I have used, I have obtained their consents.

Nurse Talk:

Throughout the book I've integrated "Nurse Talk" which offers the reader an explanation of some medical and nursing terminology. It is denoted by the icon and a reference number. Please refer to Nurse Talk explanations beginning on page 297.

INTRODUCTION

As an oncology nurse for a large portion of my career, I thought I knew about the cancer experience. I'd helped many patients maneuver through the harsh effects of treatment. Cancer was an enemy that invaded their bodies, and they needed to go to great lengths—surgery, chemotherapy, radiation and sometimes a grueling bone marrow transplant—to kill it. They suffered, and their road to recovery was arduous.

Working with them, I felt like a soldier on the battlefield fighting for my patients' wellbeing. They taught me the importance of helping people at one of the most difficult and vulnerable times in their lives. I was amazed at their incredible spirit of survival.

As connected as I felt to my patients, I didn't fully comprehend the courage it took to confront cancer every day or realize the mental, emotional, spiritual, and physical turmoil involved until I became one of them.

Chapter 1

LESSONS

I stood at Edith's bedside, glancing at the vanilla-colored slatted blinds framing the window. Gray clouds mirrored the cold inside her hospital room. Dark brown carpet, beige walls, and the tan blanket covering her reinforced a dismal day.

Her fragile, pale hands felt soft and cold as I brushed my fingers over them. Her veins, coiled and purple with age, looked like tree roots, accentuating her years and the complexity of her circulatory system. Her head was elevated, cushioned by two pillows, and her mouth gaped open, covered by a stiff plastic oxygen mask. The sound of her breathing was coarse as the airflow streamed inward, frightening me.

I moved closer to her face and gazed at Edith's closed eyelids. I noticed her sparse eyelashes looked moist. She'd closed the world out; her mind, body, and soul were preparing for her departure. She was dying of cancer.

"Edith, can you hear me?" I asked loudly. I suddenly felt silly. Of course she could hear me. She just couldn't answer. Nursing school had taught me that even coma patients can hear what is being said.

I sighed and looked out the window at the rainy mid-January afternoon. Depressing. I consoled myself with a cleansing breath, exhaled and said a prayer for Edith's soul. She was the first dying patient I'd taken care of since becoming a registered nurse. Plastered on the front of her chart was a label that read, "Do not resuscitate." Regardless of my gloominess, I wanted to provide her with as much care and compassion as possible through her last moments of life.

Edith's waist-high bedside table was covered with nursing necessities. There were suction catheters in packages, a bottle of saline, and stacks of diapers and blue pads in case she needed to be changed. A withered white rose stood in a simple vase at one end of the table. A hospital maintenance man had brought it to her one week before, when she could still offer us her charm.

I touched her shoulder, feeling the softness of her pink silk pajama top embossed with her initials on the pocket. I smiled, recalling her refusal to wear a hospital gown. She didn't need one. I thought back to the first time I'd taken care of Edith a year earlier, when I was a student nurse.

I had walked into her room wearing a starched white uniform. "Good morning, Edith. My name is Christine and I'm a student nurse. I need to take your blood pressure."

"Hand me my suitcase," she demanded. "It's in the closet."

"Sure." I opened the double door and pulled out an old, rock-hard beige suitcase the size of Alaska. "This thing's pretty heavy."

I lugged it toward her bed and carefully placed it on top of the brown woven blanket. The case was plastered with colored stickers from around the world: Belgium, France, Egypt, Japan, Singapore, and many more exotic places.

"How do you carry this around?" I asked, standing over her petite five-foot frame as she fluffed her pillow.

"Honey, I don't do the lugging," she said with a grin. Handling the suitcase as if it were a briefcase, she released the brass locks with her thumbs, making a clacking sound.

She hunched over the suitcase and rummaged through clothing and possessions. Her arms showed brown age spots, and arthritis had enlarged her knuckles. She had blue eyes and an attractive face with wrinkles in the right places. The wrinkles added dimension, as if she were a sculpture that visitors would want to see.

"Looks like you've been to a lot of interesting places," I said while watching her lay out an African-looking wooden beaded necklace on the bed.

Edith looked up at me. "I've paraded around the world many times on cruises." She lifted a royal blue kimono out of the case. "Traveling keeps me calm."

This glimpse into her lifestyle fascinated me. "Who do you go with?"

"I go on my own." She placed the kimono on the bedspread. "It's the best way to meet fascinating and famous people." She winked.

"Wow. Sounds like you've had quite an adventurous life."

Suddenly, I grew aware of the need to get my task done and move on. I picked up the blood pressure cuff housed on the wall behind her bed and motioned for her to sit in a chair.

"It's not over yet," she exclaimed.

I smiled, amused by her independent nature. Her polished attitude and confidence intrigued me.

Edith sat in the one large chair in the room and stuck her arm straight out. I took her blood pressure. "What's your next exciting destination?"

"I haven't figured it out yet." She frowned. "I need to get through the surgery first."

Edith had never married and had no children. Yet, she didn't appear lonely. She'd been in and out of the hospital throughout the past year, I'd been told. Yet, she seemed unafraid. I loved her radiant confidence, something I lacked. I wanted to learn more about her intriguing life and how she developed her self-assurance, but felt the pressure of taking care of other patients and nursing tasks.

I walked to the doorway. "I think you're a very interesting lady, Edith."

"Honey, let me tell you something. Don't let people tell you how to live your life." She sorted through more contents of her suitcase. "There's all kinds of nonsense chatter in the world." She gave me an intense look. "Sometimes hard decisions are the right ones, no matter what anyone else thinks."

I now sat next to Edith on her hospital bed. The snore-like rattle of her breathing sounded dreadful, and the dramatic rise and fall of her chest startled me. Her non-rhythmic respirations, gave me a feeling of uneasiness. Her tongue and lips were dry.

I grabbed a green toothete sponge on her bedside table and dunked it in a cup of water. Lifting her oxygen mask, I smelled her sour breath and gently moistened her mouth and lips. Her cheeks were sunken, skeletal, her facial features flat. Her once shapely body had dwindled due to cancer metastasis.

I held her hand and noticed how cool it was. Her nail beds were pale. It saddened me to see her sassiness had withered and that she had no more personality to express to the world. I wondered what she was feeling, if she could feel anything at all. How had she felt battling cancer?

I shook myself out of these thoughts and said, "You're such a special lady, Edith." My throat thickened and I welled up with tears. "I loved hearing about your exotic travels." I caressed her stiff gray hair. My voice quivered. "Edith, it's okay. Go be with God. Be at peace."

I stood, exhaled deeply, and put on the armor of emotional calmness before darting out of the room. Throughout my first year as an oncology nurse, I'd been up close with disease and suffering. I'd learned to become flexible and adaptable with my mind-set and emotions. After all, I still had to get things done.

I gathered my mental fortitude and focus, and moved quickly down the hall to check on my other patients. After finding them well, I rushed back into Edith's room. Just as I entered, she took one last heaving gasp of air.

My heart pounded as I cried out, "God bless you, Edith!" I said a prayer for her soul and watched her body collapse into relaxation.

I summoned the doctor. Upon re-entering Edith's room with the physician, a burst of warmth and tranquility came over me. He removed his stethoscope from around his neck, listened to her heart, and pronounced her dead.

Raindrops pelted the glass. I suddenly felt an overwhelming peace. Edith had made it to her final destination. I was happy to help her on this journey. My questions about how she felt during her illness weren't answered. They never would be. However, I knew whatever Edith had suffered in her battle with cancer, serenity now filled her.

Little did I know that thirteen years later, I would be in the same shoes as Edith, fighting the merciless beast.

Chapter 2

ENLISTING

I walked toward the entrance of the cancer hospital, clasping my plastic RN photo badge onto the lapel of my white uniform. It was 6:45 a.m. and the sunny April day was coming to life. As I passed the scenic fountain, droplets splashed onto me and I heard the soothing sound of cascading water. I took in the precious moments of beauty and smiled to myself, remembering how nervous I was the first time I had stepped onto these grounds as a nursing student.

I exited the congested freeway and drove slowly through the suburban neighborhood streets toward the cancer hospital. It was the first day of my senior student rotation. Insecurity and fear gained its momentum, impinging on me like the light fog that permeated the air. I raised my elbow and peered down at my white uniform sleeve, seeing my nursing school patch. As if I didn't feel awkward enough being a student nurse. It was publicized. I glanced at myself in the rear-view mirror. I was conservatively put together, my light brown shoulder-length hair in a ponytail, my crisp white-collared uniform pressed neatly. My nude make-up attempted to cover adolescent acne reborn through nursing school stress. While hospital-ready on the outside, I wasn't sure how prepared I was on the inside. Nerve-wracking questions filled my mind: *How could anyone work at a cancer hospital? Isn't it depressing? What am I supposed to say to cheer up my patients? Will they all be crying?*

I drove toward the parking lot entrance, tense, yet amazed at the acres of emerald green grass and abundant pine trees lining the campus. It looked more like a golf course than a hospital. While pulling into the driveway, I noticed a magnificent fountain. I smiled, having expected a dreary building and miles of concrete. My tension eased and I marveled at the beauty of the place. Maybe this hospital would surprise me.

That was over a year ago. Now, I sat at the nurse's station, listening to the night-shift-taped report while jotting down information about my patients. I was thankful I wasn't a student anymore. It was nice not having instructors critiquing me, nor papers to write, and I liked the camaraderie of other nurses. But more importantly, I enjoyed working with cancer patients. Their unique medical problems and personalities always made my shifts interesting.

While leaning on the medication cart, I scribbled down my patients' medication times and when to administer them on my "brain" (what a nurse calls the paper on which she keeps her written patient information). It was 7:30 a.m. The hallway lights were dim and quietness filled the unit except for the buzz of a patient call light at the nurse's station. I marched down the hallway, my nursing shoes thumping on the brown carpet. I stopped outside room 212, my turquoise stethoscope draped around my neck. I pulled my "brain" out of my pocket, and scanned the details about a young man named Justin. I hoped he wouldn't sense my unease.

The two-bed room had a tan tile floor and checkered brown and beige curtains, used to partition the patient spaces. Open vertical blinds overlooked a garden of ferns. While walking toward the window, I saw a tall, athletic guy sitting up in bed, flipping through a *Rolling Stone* magazine. I moved slowly toward him and my gaze met his. I introduced myself, noticing his boyish face, matted down hair, and long eyelashes. He was twenty, only four years younger than me. He'd had an orchiectomy–a testicle removed due to testicular cancer. [1]

Insecurity filled me knowing I needed to check his surgical area. Not wanting him to detect my apprehension, I put on my confident nurse-face. "You an early riser?" I asked with a smile.

"Nah, not normally." He placed the magazine open-face on his spread-covered thighs. "Gotta love the comfort of a hospital bed."

"Nothing like the coziness of home." I put a plastic cover on the thermometer. "How ya feeling?"

"Pretty good," he said, raising his tongue so I could insert the thermometer.

I finished checking his vital signs. "I need to look at your dressing and make sure everything's okay."

He sighed deeply. I could relate. I lifted the covers. Thankfully, the dressing was dry and showed no bleeding. As I recovered him with the blanket, I tried to lighten up the moment. "We're always asking to look at people's private parts. Pretty annoying, huh?"

An embarrassed giggle came out of him. His self-consciousness relieved me, as did his words: "Hey, you gotta do your job."

The conversation quickly changed to his plans for college and things he liked to do. "I'm in a rock band and play the drums." His freckled fingers imitated drumming in the air.

"That's really cool," I said, removing my stethoscope from behind my neck to listen to his lungs. "Music makes life better, doesn't it?"

"Absolutely!"

"Let's walk down the hallway and get you moving."

We strolled the corridor, his IV pole part of our walking trio. A smile filled his face, giving me the impression he enjoyed our conversation.

"I don't play a musical instrument, but I like to dance," I said.

"You're probably into country dancing?"

"No, that's not really my style. I like rock or club music."

"I'm not much of a dancer. Typical guy, right? Last time I checked," he said with a snicker.

We both laughed. "Yes, it definitely seems you are."

I was in awe at how upbeat Justin appeared as he dealt with his cancer. He maintained a happy-go-lucky attitude in the midst of adversity.

Not all patients were as easy to work with as Justin. Some lived with terrible physical deformities because of cancer.

Consequently, they suffered from depression and were very angry at their circumstances.

I sat cross-legged in the nurse's station, hovering over a thick blue chart, charting the details of my patients' day. I looked at my watch: 11:30 a.m. Nurse Glenda passed by, wearing a red bow in her hair.

"Glenda can you help me get Enrique up in his wheelchair?"

"Sure."

I headed toward Enrique's room, tense and fearful. I hadn't become accustomed to seeing a twenty-something man without legs or hipbones.

I knocked hesitantly on the opened door. As I walked into his room, I felt insecure, hoping I wouldn't say the wrong thing or make him angry. I wanted his world to be filled with some sense of normalcy. "Enrique, Glenda and I are here to get you ready for lunch," I said.

His room was dark, the blinds shut, television off. He lay on an over-sized blow-up bed that made a humming noise, with hoses attached at the bottom mattress. Enrique's routine was to sit in his wheelchair once a day, a task that required two nurses. Stacks of running magazines lay on a shelf next to his bed. It made me sad to see them. There were no decorations in his room, and he wore his dark hair in a military cut. I was told that he'd wanted to join the Marines before contracting cancer.

"Let me put the wheelchair next to your bed," I said.

All the staff knew that Enrique didn't want to talk before he was in his wheelchair. There was no idle chitchat allowed. He wouldn't stand for it.

His face grew intense and determined as he mentally prepared for the move. He seemed to look through Glenda and me. When I pulled the trapeze handle down from the metal rod that hung over the length of the bed, it jingled. He seemed not to notice.

He reached up. I helped raise his torso to meet the trapeze, and Glenda swung his stump to face the side of the bed. The room remained quiet except for our discussions related to the transfer. "Okay, on a count of three we're gonna move you," I said in a calming tone, wanting him to feel secure.

We lowered him into a beige bucket on the seat of the wheelchair. Even a normal sitting position was impossible for him without this device. He situated his torso comfortably in the bucket and leaned back.

Calmness spread across his face. "Take me to the patio," he said in a matter-of-fact tone. He ordered one of us to hand him his baseball mitt. Glenda squeezed his shoulder and exited the room. I wheeled him out. The sun was bright, and puffy clouds moved slowly across a blue sky.

"I'll bring your lunch," I said, hoping to spark some sense of delight in him.

After gathering Enrique's food and a few things I thought he might like, I walked outside. With closed eyes, he was enjoying the sun's warmth. I placed a baseball on the table next to him and a baseball cap I'd found in his room. I set down the tray piled with the cheeseburger he'd ordered.

I'd been told one of the doctors would stop by at times and throw the ball to him. As I stepped inside, my heart bled for this young man. I'd never seen anything like what he was dealing with. No matter how prepared I tried to appear on the outside, his situation confused me on the inside.

The destruction that cancer leaves doesn't make sense. Sometimes in the cancer battle, there are casualties that leave a person handicapped for life.

Chapter 3

Things Submerged

Thirteen Years Later

I trudged up the staircase to my second-level condo, holding onto the white wooden banister while pausing to admire the garden beds below. The snapdragons were in bloom. I was grateful to be getting home from my second job at the outpatient surgery center. My regular full-time job was in the emergency room. Since graduating from nursing school, I'd worked oncology for almost eight years and had specialized in bone marrow transplant. However, I liked diversifying my career as a traveling nurse, Post Anesthesia Care Unit (PACU / recovery room) nurse, and ER. Throughout my patient encounters, no matter what specialty, I had often taken care of people dealing with cancer. They would always occupy a special place in my heart.

The temperature rose to seventy-five degrees on the warm Thursday spring evening. My boyfriend, Skylar, waited with white roses and a bag of Chinese take-out – his Thursday night ritual for the three weeks we'd been dating ... again.

"Hi beautiful! How was your day?" he asked with a wide smile, his perfect teeth showing. He was growing silver with sandy brown sideburns.

"I'm tired, but I'm glad to see you." I gave him a kiss. "Thanks! You're always so sweet to me. Flowers *and* dinner?"

I was surprised at how tired I felt. After all, the surgery center work was much easier and less stressful than a twelve-hour emergency room shift. However, I wasn't about to let my fatigue ruin my evening with Skylar.

We went in and I kicked off my black clogs in the entryway, put the flowers in a vase and brought out dishes to the round, glass dining table.

"Ya know, you don't have to keep yourself so busy all the time," Skylar said in a fatherly tone as we sat at the table.

For an instant, I thought of our twenty-year age difference. "I know, but it's all good busyness." I liked his loving concern. "Oh and by the way, before you and I got back together, I was planning to do the Rosarito-to-Ensenada fifty-mile bike race with some guy friends in Mexico."

"You always like to be the girl about town, going, going, going," he said, dishing Kung Pao Chicken onto our plates. "Fifty miles doesn't sound like my idea of fun, but of course, I am a smidgen older than you." He cocked his head to one side and smiled, accenting the crow's feet near his eyes.

"It's a challenge. Something I've never done before."

He took my hand in his. "I trust you and support whatever it is you want to do."

"Thank you." I gave his hand a squeeze.

I walked to the kitchen and brought out glasses filled with water. "One thing my patients taught me: you never know what's gonna happen in life, so live now."

He looked at me with tender eyes. "I'm really smitten with you." He leaned in for a kiss. "I've never met anyone like you."

"Ahhh. That's so sweet." I gave him a coy smile. "And I've never met a more caring and sensitive man than you."

After we kissed, I leaned back in my chair, thinking how wonderful it was that I seemed to be one of his life priorities. "You're my calming influence."

"Let's eat, then I'll rub your feet," he said with a wink.

I sighed deeply. "Wonderful."

I'd met Skylar in August, the year before, while waiting for a male friend who was late picking me up at the Solana Beach train station in North San Diego County. On the ride down, tears over a boyfriend break-up spilled from my eyes. I sopped them up with a full package of tissues and stuffed the fallen remnants of my relationship into my purse. This was one of many boyfriend break-ups in my turbulent dating history. Why was it so hard to meet the right guy? Sick of dealing with so much heartache, I was glad to be meeting a guy friend, someone with no relationship expectations. As I stood waiting for my friend, Skylar had walked up to me and we'd started chatting. He was charming and easy to talk with. He made me laugh. In a goodbye handshake, Skylar had slipped me his number.

We sat on my white futon couch after dinner and Skylar rubbed my feet. I reclined comfortably onto a pillow and gazed at his distinguished-looking profile. I was happy to be with him, again.

"This is exactly what I need tonight," I said, looking at Skylar's dominant nose, tanned face, and manicured hair a speckled gray and sand-brown. I thought about our dating history which had had some tumultuous times. Eight months prior we were in a committed relationship which lasted six months. During that time, I was unable to get over my doubts and mind-flipping struggle in dealing with his past. Skylar's three ex-wives, two kids under the age of twelve, and lack of desire to have more children scared me. We broke up.

I dated other men, but no one as special as Skylar. He had a confident ease and loved being my cheerleader. My thinking changed. *Maybe dating an older man was a bonus.* This wasn't the life plan I had envisioned, but maybe I needed to allow it to work.

Skylar completed my foot rub, wrapped me in his arms, and kissed my forehead. "This is right where I want to be," he said.

Secure in his warm embrace, I was filled with happiness. I dismissed the thoughts of marriage, having children together, and how it would all turn out.

Days later, I hovered over maps sprawled on my white-carpeted living room floor. Feeling their smooth, thick texture, and seeing the names of European cities, added to my anticipation of taking a one-month trip to Spain and Portugal with Skylar.

"How about we fly into Madrid and spend a couple days there first?" I asked.

Skylar sat on the couch scratching his five-o'clock shadow. "Great. Let me look up the Eurail schedule to see what cities the train can take us to after Madrid."

With a cup of coffee in one hand, he peered into the booklet, his glasses resting on his nose, so intellectual and handsome. "How about Salamanca, then Portugal?"

I buried my face into the guidebook. "Wow! It's an old university town with cobblestone streets and a famous Plaza Mayor."

As I read, the names and snippets of the cities we would be visiting excitement filled me. We mapped out our itinerary, which included Lisbon, Porto, Barcelona, Sevilla, and Ibiza. The lure of a foreign land had always enticed me, but I had a gut feeling this trip would be memorable.

"Sounds like we're ready for a once in a lifetime adventure," he said. He sat on the carpet next to me and gave me a hug. I felt happy and secure...nothing could go wrong.

A week later, I was shaken from a deep sleep, feeling as if hot embers blazed inside me. I threw off my covers and realized my upper body was soaked with sweat. I sat up, shook my head, and wondered what the hell was happening. I was too young for hot flashes. Seconds after I awoke feeling like I was burning up, I shivered with cold. The entire night was a game of on-again, off-again with the pink sheet and thin white blanket. Maybe I was just working too much?

I walked to the bathroom sink, and scooped soothing cold water onto my face. Looking in the mirror, I saw dark circles under my eyes. I headed back to bed and glanced at the clock: 4:30 a.m. As I lay back down, I reflected on my activities that night. I'd gotten home at midnight after having fun with friends, going to dinner, and barhopping. Maybe I just needed a good night's sleep.

Several weeks later, I stepped into my bathtub-sized shower, beginning my routine of getting ready for my ER shift after attending a morning spin class. Plumes of steam rose above the spray of water pouring from the showerhead. I tiptoed into the water, allowing its heat to drench me. Grabbing the white nylon netted ball, I applied some shower gel and started rubbing it over my body. The aroma of cherry permeated the shower stall. I scrubbed my tanned feet and rubbed the ball up my left leg, spreading tiny white bubbles from my toes to my upper thigh.

When I reached my left groin, I stopped. A golf ball-sized lump protruded from there. Startled, I fearfully rubbed my hand over it. *What the heck?* I couldn't believe it was so large. *Creepy.*

I bent closer and touched it again as the water cascaded over my body. It didn't hurt. How weird.

I toweled off and walked into the brightly lit bathroom, then stooped forward to look at the bulging mass. I felt it again. It was rubbery and soft, not painful, but disgusting.

Fear gripped the pit of my stomach, my heart raced, and I felt as if I suddenly were going to unravel. *Oh God.*

Standing upright, I took a deep breath and pushed the negative thoughts aside knowing I had to get ready for work. Maybe it was just some sort of cyst or the start of an infection? Who knew what it was? I saw weird things in the ER all the time.

I stepped into my blue scrub pants, pulling them over the lump. I submerged my sense of panic. *Don't go there.* I had other things to think about. I finished dressing, headed out the door, and buried my fear. I'd ask one of the ER docs at work what he thought. Worrying wouldn't do me any good.

At the hospital, ER clerks were gathering insurance information and identification essentials from patients, and applying wristbands to their arms. Nurses, doctors, and techs scurried to keep pace with the demand of incoming patients. In spite of the hurried tempo and my uneasiness about the lump, I managed to remain calm and focus on my job. But I'd decided I would find Dr. Natase, otherwise known as Dr. Nice, as soon as there was a break.

I started my shift at 11:00 a.m. I walked by the central board, where the charge nurse wrote patients and doctors names, and patient diagnoses. What a relief to see Dr. Nice's name on the board, even though he wasn't assigned to my pod (section of the ER). It was late afternoon, and so far, no break in sight. I hoped my opportunity to talk with him wouldn't slip by. With the medics bringing in patient after patient, it looked like I'd have to keep my problem to myself.

Mr. Tinsely was a 90-year-old man who came from a convalescent home. The staff said he'd fallen out of bed. As he lay on the white-sheeted gurney, a gauze bandage on his left arm, spots of blood seeped through. The medics had applied the arm dressing and told me he was very hard of hearing and didn't answer questions.

"Mr. Tinsley, I'm going to listen to your lungs and take a look at you," I yelled into his hairy ear.

His cloudy gray eyes stared forward as if my words weren't penetrating. I shined a flashlight into them, checking his pupils; they were responsive, a good sign. His body was skeletally thin, the skin translucent and scaly. I lifted his hospital gown, noticing adult diapers and the musty smell of age. He lay in a permanent fetal position. A urine bag (Foley catheter) hung from the side of the gurney. When I inspected the plastic tube, I saw urine the color of orange juice with thick stands of mucus floating in it. I obtained a specimen cup, filled it with a sample, and quickly capped it, shutting out the putrid odor of ammonia. I labeled it and sent it off for testing.

Nurse Vanessa worked with me in our pod. She was a buxom, loud brunette who wore cherry-colored glasses. Twenty years of ER work had given her a great wealth of information. I always appreciated her wisdom and expertise, but not necessarily her barking demeanor.

Her eyes were fringed with lashes heavy with black mascara, and her freckled face looked intense. "Christine, the charge nurse told me the medics are bringing in a comatose overdose case," she yelled. "Get the NG tube (nasogastric tube- inserted through the nose and into the stomach) and charcoal!"

"Sure," I said, shrinking from her harsh tone. I ran to the supply cart and quickly returned to our pod.

Dr. Baxter was at the bedside before the patient arrived. He was an abnormally tall, frizzy-haired ER doctor in his fifties. No matter the situation, he always remained calm and even-tempered.

Two paramedic firefighters escorted a gurney to our pod, carrying a young twenty-something woman. A heavy-set medic hand-pumped the Ambu bag that breathed for her.

"This is a twenty-two-year-old female who was found unconscious by her roommate," the stout, dark-haired medic said. "The roommate said when she left for work at 10:00 a.m., Kendal was home, partying with friends. They were doing cocaine, ecstasy, and drinking." He helped me move her onto the bed. "The roommate came home in the afternoon and found her unconscious."

Kendal had platinum shoulder-length hair, pale skin, cobalt blue eye make-up smeared near her eyes, and black eye liner. Her petite face looked bizarre with the breathing tube sticking out of it.

The respiratory therapist immediately connected her up to the ventilator. The machine expelled a loud beep. Dr. Baxter gave orders while Vanessa and I quickly hooked up Kendal to the EKG monitor, started another IV, and inserted a nasogastric tube down her nose. Vanessa began her head-to-toe assessment while I fetched the charcoal.

This was my first overdose case, and I was unsure how to administer the charcoal. I hurried back to Vanessa with the tube of charcoal. She was labeling lab specimens at the portable desk. "Can you please tell me the best way to give this?"

Vanessa reached into a drawer of the portable nurse desk and pulled out a large syringe, slamming it on the plastic desktop. "It's gonna be gooey, so draw it up in the 60cc syringe and push it into the NG," she said, clearly irritated at me. I bypassed her attitude while listening to her instruction, even though my stomach tumbled with angst. "Since we don't know how much of the drugs she took, Tom is estimating, so he wants fifty grams followed by two-hundred-and-fifty milliliters of water."

For an instant, I pondered why some co-workers needed to have attitude. "Thanks, I'll bring it right over," I said, watching Vanessa carry a Foley catheter tray to the bedside. While emptying the tube of charcoal into a container, relief filled me as Dr. Nice walked in my direction. He was slightly overweight, and had a smooth dark moustache. I liked his caring, genuine nature.

"Oh, my gosh. Hi," I said, panicked. "I *really* need to talk to you, but I can't right now."

I glanced at the goopy contents and drew some of it up into a syringe. I was deflated, knowing how precious the random minutes of chatting with a co-worker were.

"I'll be here till eleven," he said, passing by.

I rushed to Kendal's bedside and began pushing the charcoal into the NG tube. Sadness gripped me as I watched the black contents pour into her. Such a young, pretty girl would now have to fight for her life and then battle addiction. It didn't make sense. Why had she done that? After sending the charcoal and water through the tube, I walked to the portable nurse's cart to complete my charting and talk with Vanessa.

"Sad case," I said.

"People do stupid things."

Her harsh remark took me aback, but she was right.

Fifteen minutes later, I said to Vanessa, "I'll go check the computer to see if her labs are available."

I walked toward the computer area and saw Dr. Nice. "What's up, Christine?" he asked with a wide smile, his moustache covering some of his upper lip.

I looked into his blue eyes. "I need talk to you about a personal issue." Even though I liked a lot of doctors, Dr. Nice was the one with whom I felt most comfortable sharing my symptoms.

"Okay, no problem."

"This morning I found a golf ball-sized lump in my left groin that sprang up out of nowhere."

"Does it hurt?"

"No."

"Hmmm." He crossed his arms and eyeballed the floor. "I'm not sure what it is, but I think you should have your primary care doctor further examine you."

"Thanks. That was my plan."

I squeezed his arm, relieved I didn't need to be admitted right that second. I sat down at a computer and switched gears to my patients' issues. Nursing had taught me the need to be focused and not allow worry to preoccupy my thoughts.

The next day, I made a doctor's appointment for the following week and put it out of my mind.

A week later, in Dr. Dennis's office, I sat on a comfortable burgundy chair. It looked antique with its fancy wooden back. Teal love seats sat in the corner. They seemed more suitable for an upscale house. I was uneasy and worried about the lump, and anxious to get an answer.

I glanced at the clock above the receptionist's desk and file folders: 4:00 p.m. Certainly, I was the last appointment of the day. An elderly gentleman and his wife had just been called into an exam room, leaving me alone in the waiting room. I wiggled my crossed leg with anxiety, and then decided to use this time to focus on my exciting, fun-filled travel plans.

I pulled out a piece of paper and a pen from my purse and wrote down items I needed to pack for Spain and Portugal. I also jotted down things I'd need to take to Mexico for my bike race. Finishing my lists, I looked at the rectangular glass table in front of me. A *Condé Nast Traveler* caught my eye. I flipped through it, admiring the picturesque Italian countryside. I was always open for a visual getaway, even by magazine.

"Christine," the nurse called.

I got up, gathered my purse, and headed to the exam room. It was small, simple and smelled of rubbing alcohol. Normally, that odor didn't faze me, but now I noticed it. I changed into a patient gown and sat on the paper-covered, hard orange exam table with my arms crossed, attempting to warm up in the cold room. The sink was directly across from the table, and the counter held jars of alcohol wipes, cotton balls, and thermometer covers. It was quiet except for the muted voices in the next room. *I couldn't work in a doctor's office—too boring,* I thought. I liked more excitement in my work life.

Dr. Dennis had been my internal medicine doctor for three years. He reminded me of the cartoon character Ziggy, with his large, bald head that sat on his out-of-proportion body. I liked that he was mellow and approachable. His office sat across the street from the hospital, and I would occasionally see him in the ER admitting one of his patients.

"Hello, Christine," he said in his gentle way. "What's going on with you today?"

"Well, I have a lump in my left groin that sprang up out of nowhere," I said in a nonchalant tone.

"How long have you had this?" He motioned for me to lie back on the table and palpated (feel with fingers) my left groin.

"I first noticed it in the shower last Thursday," I said, feeling nervous as he touched it.

"Does it hurt?"

"No, that's the weird thing. It doesn't."

"How are you feeling otherwise?"

"I have night sweats occasionally and am a little tired, but I'm an ER nurse, so I have reason to be tired. Right?" I laughed an awkward laugh.

"Sure." He completed his assessment by listening to my heart and lungs, and palpating under my arms and neck. "I don't know what it is, but I want you to see a surgeon," he said calmly. "What surgeon do you want to see?"

"Surgeon? What?" I swallowed hard.

"Yes, a surgeon needs to take a look at the lump."

I was dismayed. "Okay," I said, gaining my bearings. "I'd like to go to Dr. Kelsey."

I remembered sitting with Dr. Kelsey in the hospital cafeteria, sharing stories of fun trips we'd each been on. I'd taken care of many of his post-op patients in the PACU. At least I had the inside scoop on knowing lots of doctors, I thought.

"Great. I'll get his report, then we'll go from there," Dr. Dennis said.

"Thanks."

I left the office. *Another thing to take care of.* Then I turned my focus to my upcoming trips. It was better to think about happy things instead of worrying about what I didn't know. I made an appointment with Dr. Kelsey for the following Wednesday.

A week later, I sat on the hard exam table, wearing a patient gown, and waiting for a doctor. I was curious and a little scared about what Dr. Kelsey might say about the lump.

Staring at the eggshell-colored walls, my mind drifted to the details of my trips. I would leave that Friday for Mexico, and return home to California on Sunday. The next day, off to

Spain! My goal was to get an answer, end this doctor's visit, and move on.

Dr. Kelsey came into the exam room, wearing a white lab coat over his dress pants, white shirt, and blue tie. "What brings you into my office? Shouldn't I be seeing you in the cafeteria?" he joked.

His carefree personality came with a cheeky smile that left me feeling cared for and comfortable.

"I have something I need you to look at," I said, talking calmly but feeling unsettled. "Two weeks ago, a large lump appeared in my left groin all of a sudden. It's not painful. It's really weird. I don't know what it is."

I lay back on the exam table, watching him rub his hands together for warmth before touching the lump. I stared at the top of his gray hair spiked with hair gel. He palpated my lump and said, "I need to take a biopsy of it in surgery."

That annoyed me. "Are you serious?"

"Yes. I can't tell what it is without a biopsy."

"Do you think it's a cyst?" I pleaded.

"I really can't be sure until I get a sample of it," he said.

"Okay, but I'm leaving on a trip to Spain and Portugal on Monday, so I need to have it done when I come back in a month."

There was silence for a few seconds then he said, "Well then, that's when we'll do it." He cleared his throat. "Just make sure to have an appointment lined up now so we can get it done as soon as you come back."

"Yes, I'll do that."

He closed the door as he left the room. I hopped off the table and got dressed. The receptionist scheduled the appointment, which would take place at the outpatient surgery center across from the ER.

I shut the brown door and left Dr. Kelsey's office, closing my mind on what could possibly be wrong. Time to get off this continent.

Chapter 4

Carpe Diem

One thing about time, when you feel you don't have enough, it helps you accentuate the time you do have.

Thousands of bike riders spilled into the streets of Rosarito, Mexico. I was among them in the 6:00 a.m. beach chill, wearing my spandex workout shorts, grey spandex tank top, and long-sleeved black sweatshirt. Enthusiasm filled me as I stood next to my bike and talked with my five male friends and fellow racers.

"Are you guys ready?"

"Sure. It's only fifty miles and they say it's a fun ride," blurted Tyler. "How bad could it be?"

Tyler was a friend of a friend I'd met through church, which I attended occasionally. He was a sarcastic extrovert with a muscular thin frame, blond hair, and green eyes. We'd been drawn to each other instantly as friends.

"Are you sure you can do this?" Tyler joked. "Because you can back out if you want, and drive to the beer garden in Ensenada."

"Ha! I'll bet you a beer I won't finish last in the group," I said smugly, extending my hand to offer the bet.

"Wow," he said. "You're on."

We shook hands. I hovered on my bike, ready for the race to begin. The starting gun went off, and pop music blared as bikers maneuvered through the course. None of us was a diligent racer, like the bikers who passed us. Their aggressive determination radiated the intensity on their faces. They sped past us in an instant, brows furrowed and muscular legs pumping.

"Well, guys, I guess we're not going to finish first!" I yelled.

"Who cares? I'm just looking forward to you buying me a beer at the finish," Tyler said with a snicker while riding next to me.

"Good. We have something to look forward to."

The course paralleled the ocean, passing through small towns with families lining the streets as they cheered the multitude of energetic riders.

"This is so cute," I exclaimed as Mexican children flung hard candy onto the pavement to offer encouragement. "Viva, viva, viva!" they shouted.

Thirty miles into the race, the course turned inland and escalated up a massive hill. It was brown with no vegetation and kept careening upward, with no end in sight. "They call this one the road to hell," Tyler shouted, sweat glistening off his brow.

"Does this thing ever end?" I stood to pedal and felt beads of sweat on my forehead.

"I think it's about thirty more minutes of the upward climb, then it's all downhill to the end of the race for my well-deserved beer," he said, quickly pedaling up the hill.

I stopped on the side of the road and removed my black sweatshirt, the day's warmth and exertion catching up to me.

Great. I'd forgotten to apply sun block to my shoulders and chest that were now exposed. Nothing I could do. There was no way I could survive this hill with my sweatshirt on.

I inched to what looked like the top of the hill, sweat pouring off me. This had to be the top.

But it wasn't. It switched back and continued upward. Tyler was at the top of the hill, and the other guys had passed me earlier. I continued pushing the pedals full force. No time to be tired.

I arrived at the crest, after having pedaled two-and-a-half hours thus far, feeling the cool coastal breeze, and saw the ocean churn with white caps. *Yeah! Only fifteen miles to go*! I sped down the hill, the wind blowing my hair. I inhaled the smell of the ocean, and was energized. Approaching the bottom of the hill, I pedaled ferociously. I sped past other riders and kept going. All those spin classes were paying off. I reached the forty-five-mile mark and flew past Tyler, not saying anything as I went by. I kept pedaling all the way to Ensenada, a port town known for its fun bars, bargain shopping, and mild climate.

I rode through the outskirts of Ensenada, passing pink concrete houses adorned with metal bars on the windows and shanty shacks randomly scattered among the dirt landscape. I felt sad for whoever lived there and was grateful the people were so welcoming to *gringo* bikers. Like me.

I followed some fellow racers and breezed through the finish line, feeling fantastic. "Yes!!!" *A challenge completed.* The euphoric feeling was worth tackling the grueling mountain. *If I can finish this,* I thought, flashing back to my doctors' visits, *I'm fine.*

I dismounted my bike, went into the tent area for bikers, and found four guys from our group sipping beer.

"What?" said my friend Richard, a six-foot-three, stocky thirty-something man. "Christine finished before Tyler!"

"That's right," I said proudly. "You guys doubted me, huh?"

Just then Tyler came up behind me and said in a defeated tone. "Let me go buy you a beer."

I arrived home to my condo, after two nights in Mexico, on a sunny Sunday afternoon. I hadn't really paid much attention to my sunburn, but now I felt the heat and pain on my shoulders and chest. I peeked under my shirt. Bright pink skin mirrored the areas of the tank top I'd worn during the race. As with any other sunburn, I'd just rub some aloe vera lotion on it and let the plant's magic take over. I needed to focus on getting ready for my other trip.

I called Skylar, threw my backpack open on the floor, and began packing for Europe. "So how was the race?" he asked.

"It was so much fun!" I said gleefully.

"Ready for our trip?"

"Absolutely!"

Our flight would leave the next night, so I needed to kick into gear and pack wisely, with no extraneous take-alongs.

With backpacks, passports, and a zest for adventure, we were on our way to Europe.

Madrid bustled amidst old buildings ornately decorated with black wrought iron and the fine detail of what resembled intricate lace cutouts. Amazed at the architecture, I was thrilled to finally see what I had only read about in travel books.

Skylar and I walked hand in hand, enjoying the seventy-degree weather. As we strolled, we listened to the chatter of Spaniards as they drank cappuccino at outdoor cafés. The farther we walked, the more the city enticed me with its charm.

"Let's go in here," I said, dragging Skylar into a clothing store. Beautifully colored shawls filled the small shop, with vibrant reds, turquoise, and canary yellow. "This is what the flamenco ladies wear," I said, contorting my arms and stomping my heels on the floor with dominance, to mimic a dancer.

Skylar laughed. "You're ready for your own show."

We walked many blocks until we reached Retiro Park, a large park filled with enormous trees, lavish fountains, and glorious statues of figures resembling angels.

"It's so calm and beautiful here," I said, admiring a statue the size of a tree. "You can even feel romance in the air."

Skylar pulled me close and gave me a deep kiss.

Euphoria tingled inside me. Drawing my fingers through his hair, I pulled him closer into me, feeling enveloped in our love.

Gray skies and cool temperatures welcomed us into the scenic town of Sintra, Portugal. As we felt the pull of the train veer toward the station, we admired the small town dotted with orange clay-roofed houses.

We got off the train and walked toward the depot. I inhaled the dampness after the rain. What a scent. The station was small but filled with artistry. Yellow, blue, and brown hand-painted tiles welcomed us with scenes of flowers in vases.

"Look how beautiful these tiles are," I said. "I love this town already! But before we explore, let's take a nap."

"Yep, siesta time. We've definitely adapted to Spanish ways," said Skylar, re-adjusting his backpack.

After lugging our backpacks a quarter-mile uphill, we arrived at our quaint hotel decorated with Mediterranean blue tiles embedded into the building. "This is so cute. I love the lace curtains in the window and the tiles," I said.

We entered, and I collapsed wearily into a red velvet chair in the lobby as Skylar checked us in. Room key in hand, we headed to our room.

I changed into brown cotton pajamas. Before putting my top on, I looked at my bright pink shoulders. "I can't believe I still have this sunburn," I said with disgust. "The race was two weeks ago and it's as bright as it was then."

"It's pretty weird that it hasn't faded."

"Another thing that's out of whack in me. At least it doesn't hurt," I said, trying to be optimistic but feeling a pit of fear in my gut.

We lay down on the bed, Skylar spooning me into his arms. Comforted by his love, I dismissed whatever internal chaos was going on with my body.

We sat at a beachside café, enjoying the children who frolicked in the surf. The Ibiza sky was a vibrant blue, adding to the radiance of the bright day. It was 2:30 p.m. when we finished our lunch of fish and Sangria. "I'm so relaxed," I said, taking in the beauty of the coastal brown cliffs and satisfying warmth of the sun.

"This is perfect." Skylar stretched his suntanned arms. "You know, this trip is making me see some things in my life differently."

"Really?" I leaned my elbows on the table. "Like what?"

He gazed into my eyes. "Well, something you already know is that I adore you and love you to no end."

"Yes, but I never get tired of hearing it," I said, thrilled.

"I'm realizing you haven't done the things I've done in my life, such as having a child." He looked down at his interlaced fingers then looked up at me. "I want you to know when the time is right, I'm willing."

"Are you serious?" My heart sang. "Of course, I'd want us to get married."

"That shouldn't be a problem." He leaned over the arm of his chair and kissed me passionately.

We left the restaurant, and moved to a spot on the beach. After laying out my towel on the sand, I removed my short white skirt and yellow cotton top, stretched my body out on the towel, and propped my head and shoulders up with my arms to get a better view of the ocean.

"Look how clear the water is." I inhaled a cleansing breath. Peace permeating my mind.

I glanced at my legs and bathing suit bottom. Shocked, I saw my lump sticking out next to the edge of my bikini. *Gross. No, No, No.*

I grabbed my flowered beach bag and snatched the matching purple bathing suit skirt, slipping it on to cover up my bikini bottom and upper thighs. My heart pounded with fear. *Okay, don't let this upset you.* I watched a sailboat in the distance. *There's nothing I can do.*

I took a long breath, trying to regain my vacation serenity.

I'm not gonna get freaked out, I thought, and pushed the something-is-wrong-with-my-body reminder out of my head. I focused on the sound of children laughing, and emptied myself of concern. I closed my eyes and listened to the gentle lull of the waves kissing the shore.

Peering out the small airplane window, all I could see was endless light blue sky. The vast horizon echoed my smallness in the world. Skylar sat in the stiff seat next to me, touching his shoulder to mine while holding my hand on the armrest. I felt comforted and completely in love. Our trip had been a one-of-a-kind experience that bonded us even more. I didn't want to think about heading home, but it was inevitable: we were on our way.

I tried to nestle into the uncomfortable airplane seat, wrapping a thin blanket onto my shoulders.

"I wish you would have let me upgrade us to first class," Skylar said, in his husky voice.

"It's probably cold up there too." I enjoyed him rubbing my shoulders. "We've spent enough on the trip. We don't need to spend more on that." I gave him a kiss and felt the bristles from the beard he'd grown.

"I only want the best for you."

"You always give me the best," I said, happy he was always a gentleman. "But it's not like we're rich." I elbowed him in the side. "At least I'm not." Skylar had a habit of lavishing me with fine dining and gifts, even though I had told him he didn't need to do that to win my affection.

"Hey I'm an investment advisor," he said with laugh. "I'm loaded."

I gave him a stern look. "I appreciate the offer, but all I want is for you to be with me."

"That I can do."

We spent hours on the flight reflecting on the wondrous sights of Spain and Portugal.

"So when do you have to go back to work?" Skylar asked.

"In two days." I sighed. "Back to reality."

Chapter 5

NEW TERRITORY

The afternoon mid-June sunlight filtered through the vertical blinds in the ER break room. I sat at the gray table eating my lunch and resting my feet on a chair, thoughts of our trip flashing through my mind. I wanted to hold onto my vacation euphoria as long as possible, in order to put off the post-vacation blues.

I was half-watching the television mounted on one of the walls when Tonya walked in. We had worked together in the PACU before we both transferred to the ER. She wore slightly oversized blue scrubs, and her dark hair was pulled into a ponytail. She was a kind person and trustworthy friend. Now she looked tired.

"Yeah! We get to have our break together." She hugged me. "So how was your trip?"

"Insanely fabulous."

"You look like you're on Cloud Nine."

"The back-to-work-reality hasn't completely hit me yet."

"Give it a couple of days. Then you'll feel like you've never left." She opened the refrigerator and found her lunch.

"This is actually my third shift in a row. Tomorrow I start a four-day stretch off."

"Well, I hope this high lasts for a month," she said, letting out a sigh of relief when she sat down.

We talked about my trip nonstop during our half-hour break. I loved reliving the experiences, but couldn't completely squelch the thoughts about my surgery the next day.

The sky was an eruption of bright blue and the temperature a comfortable eighty degrees. I wore a denim skirt and pink top, feeling much more inclined to head to the beach instead of the operating room. Yet there I was, driving to the outpatient surgery center with my mom. I could always count on her to be there for me, especially in trying times.

While driving past the outpatient surgery center, I felt strange and a little guilty I hadn't told any of my co-workers about my operation. It was like I was cheating on them, especially since the ER was right across the street. I wanted to keep it to myself, get it over with, and move on.

I watched people walk into the tan-colored ground-level building. "It's weird not going into work today," I said to my mom.

"I bet," my mom said. She drove to the surgery center parking lot. "Are you feeling okay?"

"I'll just be glad to get this done," I said, beginning to feel nervous.

We walked into the white building, its facade accented with concrete pillars. I checked in with the receptionist and sat on a woven chair next to Mom, filling out paperwork.

She patted my arm and offered me a self-assured half-smile. "Everything will be okay." Her kind blue eyes comforted me. All her life, she'd given love and care to our family, neighbor kids, and countless stray animals that she and my dad had adopted.

"I know," I replied, picking at my cuticles. I took a deep breath and crossed my legs. I watched my foot jiggling up and down from nerves.

The door into the interior opened. A perky nurse said, "Christine, we're ready for you to come back."

I gave my mom a gentle hug before being escorted to a small locker room, where I changed into a patient gown.

"Put your clothes in this bag. We'll give them to your mom later," the nurse said.

I wanted to roll my eyes. I knew the routine, having spoken the same words many times to patients at the outpatient surgery center.

I was ushered to the holding room populated with white-sheeted gurneys, bright lights, and nurses attending to patients. The sheer whiteness made me feel alert. Doctors wore green scrubs and surgical caps as they sat on stools, talking to patients and starting IVs. I recognized some of the nurses and anesthesiologists with whom I had worked in the PACU. I liked seeing their familiar faces.

"Please put your hair up in this cap," the perky nurse said. She handed me a blue surgical bonnet and covered me with a warm blanket. It felt strange being on the receiving end of patient care.

An anesthesiologist ambled up to my gurney. It was Dr. Albany, a colleague in the PACU. He was a jolly man with a thin nose and gold-rimmed glasses that always looked smudged. "What are you doing here?" he asked, raising his thick, wiry eyebrows.

"Well, I have a lump in my groin that Dr. Kelsey is going to biopsy." My throat tightened and my voice cracked. I cleared my throat. "I'll be glad when this is over."

He smiled. "You know what's coming. Let me start an IV on you."

"Sure. It's a little weird being on this end." My voice sounded falsely upbeat.

"We'll take good care of you."

"I know you will."

I lay on the gurney, observing other patients awaiting their operations. Then my surgeon, Dr. Kelsey, came to my side, dressed in gray-green scrubs with a gray surgical cap covering his head. His cheeky smile rose up to meet his crow's feet. "How ya feelin?"

"Okay." Uneasiness crept in. "I'm ready."

"Perfect," he said in his soothing voice.

He squeezed my shoulder and left, no doubt to talk with other patients.

Five minutes later, I was wheeled into one of the OR suites. I felt increasingly scared but focused on Dr. Albany next to me as he pushed the metal rail of the gurney. It glided quickly into the operating room. I concentrated on his slight potbelly, thick hairy fingers, and gold wedding band. He talked to me, but I didn't hear most of what he said.

"There's better ways for you to get a day off," he joked.

That snapped me out of it. "I could have picked something a little more fun," I said, glancing at his receded jaw line, small double chin, and pink complexion.

When we entered the OR, I noticed the white ceiling and brightly lit surgical suite. I was glad the room was well illuminated, but I felt like it could peer into every crevice of my fears. In the background, I heard muted voices. I knew there were instruments and machines nearby, but I didn't want to look. I stared intently at a large round lamp, similar to a satellite dish that hung from the ceiling.

"Take some deep breaths," Dr. Albany said. I focused on his gentle, drawn-out words. "We need you to slide over to the table."

"Ok...ay," I said, my voice scratchy. "Why's my voice hoarse?"

"It's from nerves."

I realized then how nervous I was.

"I'll give you something for that. You're going to feel a little burning in your IV. Now start counting backward, starting at one hundred."

My chest pounded but I closed my eyes and started. "One-hundred, nin..."

I was asleep.

I awoke from surgery to the sight of light blue and maroon checkered curtains floating on both sides of me. I lay on a gurney, admiring the brightly lit recovery room accented with a shiny white floor. The sand-colored walls gave the room a tone of wakefulness. I watched nurses walking by in floral scrub tops and solid-colored scrub bottoms. I moved my toes under the piles of cotton blankets, starting to become aware of my body. I wiggled my left hand and saw the IV was still there. I felt the weight of my hair touching the tops of my shoulders, the surgical bonnet gone. A distant IV pump beeped. All that I was seeing, hearing, and feeling seemed to be magnified.

Nurses scurried back and forth. Sometimes, they'd glance at me, then quickly look away. I thought it strange how often they went by and why they purposefully looked away, but dismissed the thought and focused on my euphoria, brought on by narcotic pain medication.

Dr. Kelsey appeared next to me, dressed in a dark blue suit, white dress shirt, and tie.

"Hi," I said in a cheery upbeat voice, enjoying my pain-medication high.

"How are you feeling?"

"Great," I said gleefully, then remembered why I was there. My euphoria quickly evaporated and my stomach tightened, thinking about my left groin area. *What had they done?*

He hovered over me, making me feel like a child. His deep brown eyes peered into mine, forcing me to stare back. A concerned look took over his face, one I hadn't seen before.

My heart began to beat fast. Anxiety gained its hold. I was frantic about what words might come out of his mouth. I cleared my throat and focused on his coffee-colored eyes.

"Christine," he said in a soft tone, "I'm very sorry to have to tell you: you have non-Hodgkin lymphoma."

Panic engulfed me. I couldn't breathe. Overwhelmed with fear, I looked down at my left groin covered by a vanilla-colored blanket. Tears filled my eyes. I felt shattered. I glanced back at Dr. Kelsey. His face had softened, allowing his eyes and attractive crow's feet wrinkles to show his concern.

"Hug me," I cried out, my voice quivering with desperation.

Tears burst from my eyes and a feeling of doom flooded me. I grabbed his green-and-blue-striped tie, pulling him closer, my primal search for comfort.

He held me gently. I felt like I was bleeding sadness as my tears fell onto his tie.

He gently pulled away and said other words I don't remember. I clenched the metal gurney, trying to absorb the news. I heard no other noises in the room as the shock swirled in my head. My mom was escorted in by a nurse.

The last thing I remember was the sight of my mom and the nurses at the foot of my gurney, crying, faces red. I was sad to see my pain ripple through others. I'd been shot down by the enemy.

Two hours later, I grabbed the white portable phone on my kitchen counter and dialed Skylar's number. Exhausted and panicked at the same time, I listened to the ringing and blew my nose from the remnants of my crying jag. My mom busied herself with organizing post-op paperwork on the kitchen counter, her eyes bloodshot from crying.

"Hello," he said in his deep voice.

I glanced out the sliding glass door. Blue sky inched its way toward darkness.

"It's me," I said, my voice filled with fear. I felt like a fragile little girl needing the comfort of a man. "I just got back home from surgery." I stopped to take a shallow breath. "I have non-Hodgkin lymphoma." I was barely able to speak the words. [2]

"Oh my God." He took a ragged breath. "I'm coming right over."

Minutes later, Skylar rushed into my condo, enveloping me into his arms. My sadness exploded and we sobbed together as we held each other. When I couldn't cry anymore, I rubbed the wetness from my face, and we sat on my futon couch. My mom sat in a wicker chair at the dining room table, crying on the phone with family members.

"They did a lymph node resection, so they took out the lump and other lymph nodes in my groin," I said, readjusting my position to lie with my leg straighter, a bulky dressing on my groin. "Now they're sending it to Sloan-Kettering for testing and confirmation." I spoke in a clinical tone of voice, even though uneasiness heaved in my chest.

"I'm gonna help you." Skylar sounded sad but determined.

My eyes welled up again, but I didn't allow the tears to escape. He made me comfortable on the couch and put a pillow behind my head. I stared at the vaulted white ceiling. "Now I need to recuperate from the biopsy, have other tests, and find an oncologist." I felt as if a fog were taking over my mind.

The three of us sat stunned. My journey "on the other side" had begun. I was a thirty-eight year old cancer patient.

Chapter 6

RECUPERATING

Cancer saw me as trying to destroy it,
so it tried to destroy me.

Days later, I lay on Skylar's couch, wearing dark blue sweats, recuperating from my surgery. I peered out the horizontal blinds and looked at the ivy-covered wall in the backyard. Though fatigued, I had more on my mind than being bothered by the heat of the summer day.

There was one person I knew in my gut I needed to call, Colin, one of my favorite former patients. He was an attractive, muscular African-American football player who had been studying pre-med in college when leukemia struck him down. I was in my late twenties when I took care of him on the bone marrow transplant unit (BMT). Some years after working on the surgical oncology floor, I'd decided to become more specialized and became a BMT nurse.

I had entered the anteroom outside Colin's isolation room and scrubbed my hands in the sink with a yellow foam scrub brush, feeling the stiff plastic bristles under my nails. I was there to give him anti-nausea medication. After stuffing my hair into a flimsy blue hair cap, I had stretched light blue booties over my nursing shoes and covered my nose and mouth with a paper mask. While donning a stiff, yellow paper isolation gown, I heard yelling.

"Can you leave?! Now!" Colin shouted, clearly enraged.

As I walked into Colin's room, I heard his father say with frustration, "Sure, whatever you want."

The six-foot-five man whisked past me. I caught a whiff of his cologne covered by the smell of cigarettes. These scents couldn't be helping Colin's nausea. A rule all oncology nurses know, and families are taught, is never to wear any perfume or cologne when with patients. Chemotherapy heightens a patient's sense of smell.

I walked straight to the IV pump, hung the mini IV bag on the pole, and programmed the pump to deliver the med. I tried to think of the right words to say.

"It sounds like you're having a bad day. Are you okay?"

Colin sat upright in the bed, arms crossed and a scowl on his face, trying to pretend this wasn't his reality. He had light skin, piercing hazel eyes, and a jagged scar on his upper forehead, which didn't detract from his handsome face. He stared silently at the television that hung in a corner of the triangle-shaped room, which was a little bigger than a large closet.

I carried the gold-colored basin filled with liquid green vomit off his bedside table and dumped the contents into the toilet. While flushing it, I was thankful I no longer gagged at this task like I had while in nursing school. After rinsing out the basin and returning it to his bedside table, I said, "Sometimes family doesn't know what to say."

Colin never looked for sympathy and was guarded about verbalizing his fear and sadness. However, anger and frustration permeated his words. The world in which he now lived was a far cry from two months prior, when he'd been playing football, living in a college dorm, and studying to be a doctor. This ambitious nineteen-year-old had flu-like symptoms and unrelenting fatigue. From the college infirmary, he was sent to the hospital for further testing, which led to his diagnosis.

"I can't stand being in here!" He threw back the sheet covering him. "I hate my family asking me how I feel all the time." His jaw tightened.

"You have every right to be angry," I said in a sympathetic tone. "This is rough."

I glanced at a framed photo on a table next to his bed. He was dressed in his football uniform, kneeling, one arm on a knee, the other cradling a football. His thick eyebrows, curly brown hair, and rugged physique were a far cry from the thin, bald teenager lying in the hospital bed. My heart ached.

Colin had been in the hospital for weeks and had received high-dose chemotherapy and total body irradiation to eradicate his defective immune system. After that, he received new bone marrow from his donor. Prior to all of this, he had been hospitalized and received chemotherapy, putting him into remission (cancer responding to treatment), which is needed before transplant.

The IV pump beeped. Colin flipped the channels with the remote, landing on a rerun of *The Munsters*. "Stupid show."

"I know this whole thing really sucks." I attempted to sound strong but felt sad for him. "It's not fair that you were in college living a normal life and now you're in here." I crouched to the level of his bed and looked up at him. "You're in a battle right now and I don't plan on you losing. I'm here to help you get through this."

He closed his eyes and his skin color slowly returned to its normal shade. I stood, walked to the door, and let out a sigh, not knowing if I was a calming influence, a mediator, or an annoyance.

On another day, I stood wearing my isolation gear in the small anteroom, holding Colin's lab work and an IV antibiotic. It was the third week of July, a week after his transplant. Knowing Colin would be disappointed with his lab results, I took a deep breath, feeling the paper mask brush my lips. I wasn't comfortable dealing with angry people. I'd have to remind him that it takes time and patience to heal. [3]

I'd entered Colin's dimly lit room at 8:00 a.m. and, finding him asleep, tiptoed toward the IV pole. I placed the lab results on his bedside table and rummaged through the top drawer of the nurse's cubicle to find an alcohol wipe. I scrubbed an area of tubing with the wipe and smelled the antiseptic. Connecting the antibiotic into the tubing, I listened to the mechanical pulse of six IV pumps running.

Colin stirred, sat up, and pushed the button for the overhead room light. He grabbed the paper. "That's it? 0.2?" He threw the paper. It landed on the tile floor near his bed. "I had my transplant a week ago. I expected it to be higher."

"Well," I said carefully, "remember the transplant process is like a garden. We replanted new marrow, and now we need to be patient as the seeds grow into a healthy plant. It takes time. This is normal."

I picked up the paper, my nerves rattled. "Do you want me to leave this in your room?"

He nodded. I placed it on the bedside table. "You gotta trust that this is part of the deal," I said. "I know it's horrible, but I believe going through all this is going to make you a better doctor later. Doctor Colin."

A look of ease crossed his face. "Time just goes so slowly in here when I'm sitting around doing nothing," he said, flipping on the television.

"What, I'm not entertaining enough for you?" I asked, moving my blue booties on the floor, imitating a shuffle.

He gave me a grin.

I was one of the few nurses who could make Colin laugh. We both had a dry sense of humor and enjoyed the heckling we gave each other. Colin didn't like most of the nurses and requested me as much as possible. I was assigned to him most days.

"I guess you're entertaining most of the time," he said as he put the television on mute. "Until you make me swallow some pills. I know you get a sick satisfaction from that."

"Oh, so now I'm sick," I said, faking a loud cry. "You really know how to flatter a girl."

"I don't need to flatter any girl," he blurted. "I've got good looks and sarcasm. All the ladies love me."

"Can't argue with that," I paused. "Keep focused on the goal, getting back to school to enjoy college life and, of course, studying to become a doctor. You gotta have it all right, good looks, sarcasm, *and* the MD?"

He laughed. "Yeah, I can do that."

I left Colin's room and removed my gown and isolation garb. Standing in the anteroom, I felt relieved, thankful for our special bond and that he liked me. His case in particular tugged at my heart strings. It was hard enough to be a teenager or young adult trying to gain a sense of who you are in the world, without adding cancer on top of it. I shook my head, thinking how scared Colin must be. One thing I knew, if this kid didn't make it, it was going to kill me.

Two hours later, Colin sat cross-legged on his bed and lifted a plastic spoon of red Jell-O into his mouth. Attempting to take a bite, he spit it into the cup and said, "How pathetic, I can't even eat Jell-O." He dumped the cup onto a Styrofoam tray on his bedside table. "Now what are you gonna try and make me do?"

"You don't need to eat right now," I said, taking the tray to the anteroom. I reminded myself that part of the emotional armor I wore to take care of BMT patients was to incorporate humor and not to take their insults or emotional upheavals personally.

I walked to the IV pole next to Colin's bed. "You're getting all the nutrients you need right now from your friends here." I gestured to the array of hanging bags that included a yellow bag called Total Parenteral Nutrition (TPN), and a white bag called Lipids.

"Just pretend these bags are your favorite food. Can I take your order?" I said, cocking my head while mimicking a waitress writing down his request. "Is it steak or a burger today?"

He looked away and gave a deep sigh.

"Time to get in the shower," I said, grabbing packages of alcohol wipes out of the nurse's cubbyhole drawer to clean his Hickman catheter before disconnecting his IVs.

"You can buy me a burger when I get outta here," he said, ambling into the bathroom to shower.

"Deal."

I removed old tubing from six IV pumps and placed new bags and tubing on the silver IV pole. It was as if I were hanging ornaments on a Christmas tree. Changing the strands of tubing reminded me of working with a string of macramé. [4]

I heard the swoosh of the closing anteroom door. Betty, Colin's mother, entered. "Is his nausea any better?" she asked, batting her thick mascara eyelashes and wearing her isolation garb. She was a Caucasian woman in her early fifties with a southern drawl. "Are his mouth sores any better?" Her mask made small movements as she asked.

"A little. He's talking more, but not eating."

"This is expected, right?" Her voice escalated to a high pitch with a hint of anxiety.

"Perfectly normal for where he is in this process. The chemo and radiation causes the mouth sores. He's still on the morphine drip."

She sat in a chair next to Colin's bed and fiddled with her wedding band.

Fifteen minutes later, Colin came out of the bathroom and plopped down on the clean sheets of the bed. "I can't believe a shower leaves me so tired," he said.

"Just rest and you'll be okay." Betty gawked at him. "It's sure hard seeing you this worn out." She shifted in her seat and the yellow gown she wore made a rubbing sound.

Colin had dark circles under his eyes, which he closed when laying down. I remained silent and began hooking up his IVs after cleaning his Hickman catheter with Betadine and alcohol.

"It's a beautiful day outside today," Betty said, her voice rising with each syllable. "I brought you some mail. Your brothers are good and..." she babbled on.

Colin raised his head off the pillow. "Stop spending so much time here!" He plopped his head back on the pillow. "I don't need your pity!"

Betty looked at me wide-eyed. She shifted her focus to the floor.

"We should let him rest for a while," I said, feeling sorry for her. I motioned for us to leave the room.

After removing our isolation gear, we met in the hallway. "I know you're understandably hurt," I said, feeling the remnants of his outburst myself. Her arms were crossed and she looked up at the white ceiling. "He's angry about this whole thing. He's in healing mode so he's going to feel exhausted."

"I never seem to say the right things." Tears filled her blue eyes. "I really try to be a good mother."

"You are," I reassured her. "It's gotta be frustrating for him to see himself exhausted after a shower, especially considering he's an athlete. Now he's stuck in the hospital, having to depend on all of us." I stroked her shoulder, feeling the softness of the light blue velour shirt she wore.

"It's not fair," she said, shaking her head, her brown curls brushing the sides of her rouged cheeks.

I gave her a gentle hug. "It never makes sense. But we're here to help you all get through this."

"I know," she said, sniffling.

"You're his mom, so most of his frustration is going to come out on you."

"All I can do is grin and bear it."

"Yes, hopefully with humor." I smiled.

We embraced and I felt Betty's body shake with grief. I was reminded that dealing with cancer is a family affair. The battle is hard on everyone.

Two weeks later, I walked into Colin's room wearing a mask and carrying a lunch tray of mashed potatoes and chicken. He had been moved to a regular single-bed room, which still had a special filtration system to eliminate germs. People who entered didn't have to gown up; they just needed to wash their hands and put on a mask before coming into the unit.

The shades were pulled, not allowing a glimpse of the hot summer day. The lights were off except for a dull overhead light. Colin sat on the side of his bed with hunched shoulders, staring at his clasped hands.

I delivered the food tray to his bedside table and sat next to him on the bed. "You look really sad right now."

He cleared his throat and gazed at his long feet. "I can't believe my life has come to this, staring at the walls of a hospital room."

I gently touched his shoulder and gave him a hug. "This is where your life is right now." I looked at his sad face. "But this isn't the end of your story."

Colin stayed silent.

"You are going to have an extraordinary life, become a doctor, and be a different person, a stronger person, because of this."

"How do you know?" he asked with a hint of sarcasm.

"I feel it. I just know." I let go of his shoulder, stood up, and pushed the tray of food closer to him. "Now your job is to eat more, walk the halls to gain your strength, and get out of here." I hunched down and looked into his eyes. "Can you do that?"

He gave me a confirming look, straightened his posture and grinned. "Someday I'm gonna kick your butt in payback."

I smiled. "Good."

I turned on the overhead light and exited the room, content. Some days, part of my job as a nurse was to be more like a motivating coach, setting goals for and making positive requests of my patients as they fought for their lives.

The following month, on another sweltering afternoon, I placed discharge paperwork and medications on top of Colin's bedside table. I glanced out of his hospital window to see enormous pine trees casting shade beneath them. The sight offered me a respite from the range of emotions I was feeling that morning. Colin and I had formed a special patient-nurse friendship throughout his hospital stay. Now it was time for me to set him free.

"You get to leave on one of the hottest days we've had this year," I said, in an even tone, trying to hide my fluctuating emotions. I was sad to see him go but delighted he could leave.

While discussing discharge instructions with Colin and Betty, I remained upbeat, grateful I'd been a part of helping him through a horrendous storm. My motherly instincts flared. I wanted to make sure he'd always be okay.

Colin stood towering over me, wearing a blue Nike oversized t-shirt that enveloped his thin frame. He no longer looked like an athlete with taut muscles. Months of illness and hospital confinement had left him lighter and weaker. But his affect was brighter. He smiled more and exuded a sense of ease.

I stared into his greenish-brown eyes, my eyes misting. Outstretching my arms like a hawk, I said, "Okay, give me a hug."

We hugged tightly. I felt a lump in my throat and knew my relationship with Colin was unique. During our embrace, deep happiness filled me, as I knew he was ready to be launched toward his life's mission.

While releasing his embrace, I looked up at his strong chin and bright face. I handed him a *Gray's Anatomy* book to help with his studies. "Go get your dream."

His mouth stretched into a smile. "There's no doubt. I will. Thank you."

Colin became a doctor, and our nurse-patient relationship turned into a friendship. He started a mentor program matching teen cancer patients with young adult cancer survivors. Colin had asked me to be a board member for his organization. I was honored and accepted, proud of all he'd accomplished, but especially grateful he was healthy. Our journey through cancer extended further than either of us could have imagined.

Now, nervously, I dialed his number. As the phone rang, I felt my energy lift.

Colin answered. "Hello," in a strong voice.

"Hi, it's Christine," I said, feeling like my old (pre-cancer-diagnosis) self until I remembered why I'd called. "I have something to tell you." I blurted, "Guess what? Your nurse has cancer."

Silence on the other end.

"I know. It makes no sense," I said uncomfortably.

"I'm in shock." He sounded depleted. "I'm so sorry." Then he switched immediately into caring mode. "You can call me anytime, even if it's in the middle of throwing up."

He had lived through the hells of chemotherapy and treatment. We both knew I would soon experience similar trauma. A sense of relief came over me. I was not alone.

Colin had gone full circle from being a cancer patient to becoming a doctor. He often came in contact with doctors with whom I worked on the BMT unit, including the man in charge of the unit.

The director looked like Clint Eastwood. Highly respected, he was well-known in the oncology field, having authored many medical books. With all his accolades, he was down-to-earth, funny, and nice.

Colin told him about my diagnosis. One day, the BMT director called and told me how sorry he was to hear of my misfortune. A call from him was like receiving a call from God. One of the most brilliant men I'd ever met had taken time out of his busy day to send me his sympathy! I felt encouraged. So much caring and compassion was coming my way.

I realized how deeply people are affected when they hear someone they know has cancer. It's like an obnoxious alarm clock that goes off, a jarring reminder that our time is limited. While moving through day-to-day life, people usually don't think about death. When someone is diagnosed with cancer, it brings up that possibility, along with many emotions and questions.

Chapter 7

JUGGLING

Mentally you try to process that life is completely different from what it was and that it would probably be different for the rest of your life.

A week later, I looked out of the automatic door of the ER entrance to a foggy morning. I sat at the triage desk in my baggy blue scrubs, taking a patient's vital signs. I'd had some days to recuperate from the surgery, and went back to work but hadn't told my coworkers or boss about my specific operation. Some knew I had a procedure and needed to be off my feet. Still sore and tired, all I wanted was to get through my twelve-hour shift.

"What is the reason you came to the ER today?" I asked the frail elderly woman stooped over in the seat across from me.

"I tripped on my kitchen rug when I was trying to give my cat his food," she said, showing me abrasions on her forearms.

"Are you in pain?"

"Yes, Honey, I'm always in pain," she said, tilting her wide-curled head to give me a smirk.

"No, I mean from the fall." I leaned sideways to look deeper into her eyes.

"My wrist hurts."

"Okay, I need you to sit in the lobby, and then we'll call you back."

My day was occupied with patients coming to the ER with a gamut of complaints. I was actually happy for the distraction from myself, and, surprisingly, remained in my normal upbeat mood. When I felt pangs of discomfort in my surgical area, I would readjust how I was sitting and take some Advil. It was a challenge to have the energy for my shift, but I had to do what I had to do.

At 7:30 p.m., my workday was finally over. Heading out the paramedic entrance, I enjoyed the warm evening air and looked up at the radiant moon rising as dusk disappeared. I was now entering another phase of my life; the upcoming months would be difficult. I didn't feel sad, but numb, indifferent.

I needed to go home and sleep. I had to keep my life as normal as possible and wrap my head around my new itinerary – the cancer patient to-do list.

The next week, I sat with my fingers interlaced in Skylar's, waiting to be called into Dr. Mahdavi's office. The oncologist assigned by the insurance company, he was also a doctor with whom I had worked on the oncology floor at a different hospital from the one where I'd started my nursing career.

As I sat in my stupor, feeling the warmth of Skylar's hand caress mine, one of Dr. Mahdavi's patients for whom I'd cared for five years earlier came to mind...

I had carried a bag of blood down the long fluorescent-lit hallway, exhaling deeply before I entered Patricia's room, an attempt to keep my sadness at bay. I knew Patricia's prognosis, as did she. Her treatment phase had ended. Her cancer hadn't responded to the many different types of chemotherapies she'd received, instead spreading to her bones. She had chosen end-of-life care, which meant she would receive care to make her comfortable, rather than aggressive treatment aimed at a cure.

Upon entering her room, I saw her burly blond husband Paul. His masculine, suntanned fingers were intertwined with Patricia's, making her hands look like those of a small child. I smiled, seeing her cradled in his comfort, and couldn't help but want that in my own life someday. I was feeling the pain of a bad relationship that had recently ended.

In a deep voice, Paul announced, "Looks like your lunch is here, Patricia."

A shy smile crossed across her sweet cherub face, her doe-like emerald eyes watching me with care. She wore a tangerine nightgown, which contrasted with her pale skin. Patricia was fifty and appeared forty. She'd been battling breast cancer for many years.

After checking her armband, I hung the blood transfusion on her IV pole and swabbed an area of tubing. While I programmed the IV pump and started the transfusion, Paul joked, "Is that the blood from the fast food place or the fine-dining restaurant?"

I grinned.

Paul adored Patricia to no end. He was by her side every day, most of the time kissing her fondly on her cheek or forehead. If he wasn't showing her affection, he was joking with the nurses.

Patricia chuckled at him. As she smiled, her bright pink lipstick was smeared at one corner of her mouth. She knew he would do anything to make the situation more lighthearted and entertaining than just have her lying in her hospital bed staring at the walls. She deserved all the love and affection he showed her. Even in illness, her light-bulb personality ignited a heartfelt adoration in all who met her.

"Come on," I retorted. "I'd only give her the best."

We all giggled. "Patricia, how ya feeling?" I asked.

"I feel tired and weak," she said in a dainty voice, I detected her Swedish accent. "I know the blood will help."

"Look at this as your energy boost for the day."

"I hope you're right," she said, squeezing Paul's hand.

"Go ahead and relax...take a nap if you'd like. I'll check on you in fifteen minutes, but call me if you need anything."

I walked down the hall to check on another patient, my sorrow lingering. This amazing lady would soon be taken away.

Fifteen minutes later, I returned to Patricia's room, cast in brightness from the afternoon sun. She was sleeping, her bald head covered with a snugly fitting pink and yellow knit cap. Paul was stroking her hand. Tears came to my eyes, but I pushed them back. I felt honored to see such a delicate, rare love displayed in front of me. As I lived with my heartache, they lived with the upcoming loss of their extraordinary love.

Now I shook off the memory, my palm moist with perspiration. I let go of Skylar's hand and repositioned myself in the chair. *That can't be my outcome,* I vowed silently. Inhaling a cleansing breath, I scanned Dr. Mahdavi's waiting room. It was small, with six brownish-mauve chairs and two wooden tables. The décor was dull and outdated, the chairs paired with pale mauve walls. I stared at an area of carpet two feet away, in a haze. I couldn't believe I had an oncologist. Skylar didn't say a word.

A smiling nurse escorted us into the exam room. She reminded me of myself when I entered a patient's room, always upbeat. My mind started to spin. When Dr. Mahdavi and I had worked together on the oncology floor, never in a million years had I imagined that someday I would become his patient.

Skylar and I sat on cushioned chairs. I looked around the room at the exam table, a jar of cotton balls, and a blood pressure cuff mounted on the wall. My mind became relaxed. The familiarity soothed me.

Dr. Mahdavi entered the room wearing a white lab coat and his usual calm persona. "This is quite a surprise," he said in his Persian accent, closing the door quietly.

"Tell me about it," I replied, rolling my eyes.

I introduced him to Skylar.

"Glad to see you're going to help her with this," the doctor said.

"I'm willing to do whatever is needed," Skylar said in a respectful tone, like an army soldier speaking with a captain.

"Goo..d," Dr. Mahdavi said and sat on a squeaky stool, propping the thin manila-colored chart onto the exam table.

"I see the report here." His brown eyes fixed on a piece of paper. "Mixed-cell follicular non-Hodgkin lymphoma." [5]

I nodded calmly for a moment, feeling like we were still colleagues, then remembering I was now a patient.

"Now we need some lab work, a CT scan, a PET scan, and a bone marrow biopsy," he said, flipping papers. "Then we'll find out what stage it is and define a treatment plan."

"Fine." It seemed nothing he said was related to me.

Dr. Mahdavi gave me a gentle hug, shook Skylar's hand, and left the exam room.

I marched swiftly out of the office, and pushed the elevator button, anxious to leave the cancer center. Skylar hovered next to me.

"We're going to do what we have to do." He put his arm around my shoulder.

I wanted to explode as I thought about taking on the life of a cancer patient. I said nothing even though I wanted to scream. I fought back tears, and stepped into the elevator.

It was a beautiful beginning of July day when I entered the nuclear exam building near the hospital. I presented myself to the front desk for my PET scan, was given forms to fill out, and sat in the lobby filled with upscale sofas. I heard a blaring news channel on a television, irritated to be listening to the latest murder report. I brushed loose strands of hair from my face and filled out the paperwork. Now my life was based on what I needed to do, not what I wanted to do.

"Christine, right this way."

A dark-haired, petite technician escorted me into a small room with a recliner lounge chair. Standing next to the recliner was a blond, thirty-something man, who looked like a weightlifter. "This is Jeremy, the technician who will be prepping you for the procedure," she said politely.

Jeremy read my paperwork. "So you work at the hospital?"

"Yeah, I'm an ER nurse," I said, proudly. "I used to be an oncology nurse."

"Wow." He sounded bewildered.

Jeremy left the room to get IV supplies and re-entered. In an upbeat voice he said, "The good thing is non-Hodgkin lymphoma has a great cure rate." He was clearly trying to cheer me up.

"Thanks," I said, trying to feel excited.

He left the room again to get the special container housing the radioactive isotope.

Jeremy wore special gloves and brought in the isotope. It was housed in a metal box that looked like something the Secret Service would carry around. A feeling of revulsion came over me when I saw the box. [6]

He told me a story about his daughter, showing me her picture on the other side of his badge.

"She's so cute," I smiled. I knew his trick: distraction.

He sat on a stool, removed the syringe from its container, and injected its contents into my IV. "Now you're radioactive. I'm gonna turn off the lights. See you in forty-five minutes." His deep voice sounded sympathetic as he departed the room.

With two blankets piled on me, I lay comfortably on the recliner in the pitch-black room that was the size of a large closet. I had been instructed to move as little as possible. My body lay quietly, but my mind was uneasy, bouncing from thoughts of, *This is crazy, I feel fine, I can't be sick,* to, *Remain calm, take a nap, and get through it.*

I'd relaxed to the point of almost falling asleep. "Christine, time for your scan," Jeremy said. He introduced me to another technician who was rail-thin with jet-black hair.

I walked into a large room, dominated by a PET scan machine that looked like a huge eggshell-colored LifeSavers candy. One wall of the room was glass, allowing remnants of the pretty day in.

Feeling intimidated, I stood in my jeans and white t-shirt listening to the instructions from the technician, smooth jazz music played in the background. "Please lie down here," she said, pointing to the sled-like platform.

Once I was lying down, she draped a blanket over my body and strapped my arms and legs close together with Velcro. "Are you claustrophobic?" she asked.

"No," I said nervously, as I looked up at the machine.

"The scan will take about forty minutes, and if at any time you aren't feeling okay, just talk." Her pale-almond face looked calm. "I'll be able to hear you."

"Okay." I took a deep breath.

"I'll have music on in the background also."

I looked up at a forty-five degree angle toward the thick LifeSavers candy-like machine, noting the small opening I needed to fit through – major confirmation I'd keep my eyes shut during the exam. The machine began making a swooshing sound, and the sled moved me incrementally into it for a test run.

My heart pounded and I took a deep gulp. I was afraid of the seven-inch closeness of the machine surrounding my head.

"Excuse me," I yelled anxiously.

The intercom came on. "Yes?"

"I need a minute." The sled moved back out, and I could hear the music again. The tech came to my side. "Just give me a minute," I exhaled, feeling as if I were hyperventilating. "I need to get my mind straight."

"Take your time."

I took some deep breaths and searched for a tactic to help get me through it. The machine made a noise like propeller blades moving. I could feel my heart pound again. *Calm down; it's okay.* I prayed, *Please God, help me through this,* even though the last couple years I hadn't prayed much. *Why do I only talk to God when I need something?*

"Okay, I'm ready."

The sled inched into the machine again, scanning sections of my body every five minutes. I kept telling myself not to open my eyes. Instead, I listened to the music, kept my body still, and found my happy place.

The beaches of Tahiti came to mind; turquoise ocean, swaying coconut trees, and vibrant white sand. I'd never been to Tahiti, but it had always been my dream place to go. Calmness took over and I was able to keep myself in a trance-like state.

After the exam was over, I walked out of the thick-walled building and into the sunny day. Relieved, I stood in the middle of the parking lot and lifted my head to the sky, enjoying the sun's warmth. In a small voice I said, "Thank you, God." I didn't want to do this journey alone.

Puffy clouds dotted blue sky, showing off another beautiful summer day. I climbed the stairs to my condo, letters in hand, and opened the door. I craved the calmness of my home. I tossed my sandals off in the entry, plunked my purse and keys on the table, and began flipping through the mail. I stopped when I saw a letter from my condo association. Irritation rose inside me. What else did they want? I'd just sent a one thousand dollar check for a mandatory special assessment fee one month before. *Why does everything have to happen all at once?*

Two condos were undergoing mold detoxification. Normally, when an association collects dues, they put reserve money in an account for emergencies. In my association, however, someone stole the money, so all owners needed to pay a special assessment fee to get the moldy condos fixed.

I let out a sigh, noticing tension in my shoulder, and bent my head to the side, rubbing a tight muscle. Maneuvering my fingers to the base of my neck, I massaged gently, until I felt two hard, dime-sized lumps. I cringed. *Oh my God!* Shock and disgust filled me. Panic gripped me at my core. I screamed. *Oh my God, the lymphoma is spreading.* I quickly moved my hand away and trembled, afraid of my body. I crouched to the floor, rolled into a ball and wept. *Why is this happening to me?*

Ten minutes later, I sat Indian-style and tried to regain my composure. I opened the letter. Unbelievable! I threw it down and called Skylar.

"I can't believe this." I said, enraged. "I'm so pissed off right now."

"What's going on?"

"The association is assessing all owners more money. Three thousand dollars!" I yelled.

"What?!"

"Yeah. I just got a letter saying another condo has major mold damage and since there's no money in the reserve fund we need to fill the gap. I don't have three thousand dollars." I was half crying. "Oh, and on top of that, I'm worse. Now I have lumps in the back of my neck!"

Skylar was silent.

"What am I supposed to do?" I screamed.

"Honey, we'll figure something out," he said calmly.

"Ahhhhh! I gotta go."

I hung up, sobbing hysterically. Nothing could console me. So many things were out of control.

One chaotic Thursday, my ER pod burst with patients needing attention. So far, I'd been able to swat away distractions, separating my work from the things I needed to do in my personal life, such as scheduling and undergoing tests. I had even quit my second job so that I could be fully present at work. I hoped I would continue to submerge the preoccupying thoughts about my physical problems so I could remain focused on my job.

Mrs. Bradley, an elderly patient, had been brought in from a nursing home. She'd refused to eat for two days and hadn't urinated in over twelve hours. She had matted down gray hair and sunken cheeks and smelled stale.

"Mrs. Bradley, I'm going to put a Foley catheter in you," I said, after explaining to her what it was. "This might feel cold." I cleansed her private parts with a Betadine swab stick.

"Owwww," she yelled.

"Sorry, I know it's uncomfortable. Take some deep breaths." I carefully inserted the rubber tube into her urethra.

Tanner, an ER tech whose spiky platinum-colored hair made him rocker-looking, came to my pod, but he couldn't see me behind the drawn blue curtain.

"Christine," Tanner called out.

"I'm in here," I said. "I'm almost done putting in her Foley."

Hazy yellow urine flowed into the bag. I placed it along the bottom portion of the gurney, disposed of the paper tray and rubber gloves, and hurried to the center of my pod.

Tanner was waiting for me with arms crossed. "What's up?" I asked, rushing to the sink to scrub my hands as he followed.

"I have a special surprise for you," he said, moving his fingers up and down his crossed arm as he mimicked playing a keyboard, a constant habit he had.

"What?" He always needed to make everything a test of my patience.

"Try and guess what I'm gonna say!" He moved his arms in a rolling motion as if we were playing Pictionary.

"I don't have time for your wise cracks today," I said, annoyed. "You're bringing me another patient?"

"Jackpot!"

With a huff, I walked past him toward an empty gurney and put a clean sheet on it.

Another nurse who worked with me, Lisa, wore her wild blonde hair pulled back by a scrunchy. When we weren't at a patient's bedside, she liked to tell me about her most recent hiking adventures. I saw her blue clogs and light blue scrubs under the closed curtain in Bed One. I was about to tell Lisa about our surprise, when over the intercom the secretary announced, "Christine, you have a phone call on line four."

"Ugh."

I rushed to the phone. It was the outpatient cancer center calling to ask questions before my bone marrow biopsy the next day. "Yes, I'm aware," I uttered into the receiver, confirming I could have nothing to eat or drink six hours before the test.

Just then, an alarm in Bed Four screeched. Lisa was still busy with a patient. I hung up the phone and ran to see what the problem was. The patient's blood pressure was elevated. I recycled the machine to take it again. "Christine, call on line five," the intercom blared.

I again rushed to the phone, frantic and increasingly upset: "Yes, this is Christine."

It was my medical insurance company. I talked on the phone while simultaneously looking and listening to what was going on in my pod. Tanner planted himself in the middle of my pod, stood with arms crossed at a distance, and looked at me curiously.

Finishing the call, I hung up the phone.

"Look at you, Miss Popular. What's up with the calls?" he asked.

"Nothing," I said, walking past him angrily, trying to focus on work.

I rushed to another patient who was yelling that he needed to go to the bathroom. I assisted him, maneuvering his IV pole along the way. I closed the bathroom door and leaned on one of the nurse's portable desks. Resting my chin on my hand, I scanned my pod and my patients lying on gurneys.

Stress raged through my body. I felt I was unraveling and having trouble concentrating. Fear gripped the pit of my stomach. *I'm sicker than my patients!*

It was time to tell my boss I needed time off.

The pulse of the ER was still chaotic, but I'd managed to wrap my head around my patients and help them with their problems. Instead of allowing myself to feel distracted, a resolve came over me.

On my late afternoon lunch break, I trudged up the back stairwell and its shiny beige concrete steps toward the office of my boss, Dominique. The echo of my footsteps made me acutely aware of my climbing efforts. When I reached the top,

I paused. *Here goes.* I reluctantly understood that from this point on, my life would be dominated by cancer. Everything would be in its time, not mine.

Dominique's door was slightly ajar. I knocked softly, watching her swivel the cushioned office chair and her thin frame in my direction. She smiled, motioning me to come in while she talked on the phone, holding it next to her neck-length, curly brown hair. She looked as if she could work in a corporate environment with her stiff white blouse, blue trouser pants, and pink pearl earrings and necklace, her signature.

I stood, feeling nervous, and tried not to listen. As I scanned the room, I saw wooden bookshelf filled with ER books. Her large metal desk was piled with stacks of papers and files. She hung up and motioned for me to sit in a chair next her.

"Can I talk to you?"

"Sure," she said, relaxing her tone from the serious business talk of a moment before.

I gazed at my hands as they rested in my lap. I rubbed my thumb against my palm, not knowing how to start the conversation. With a deep breath, I hesitated, then lifted my head and stared into her royal blue eyes. "I just want you to know I'm feeling distracted from my job."

She listened intently.

"I have cancer," I said, slowly.

"Oh my God!" Tears filled her eyes.

I voiced more specifics, feeling disconnected from my words. "The pressure of keeping it together at work while dealing with my own stuff is weighing on me," I said with relief. "I don't think I can work right now."

"Of course," she said sympathetically. She grabbed a tissue to dab her face.

"What can I do to help you?"

"I haven't told anyone yet and I can't face telling them." I tried to squelch the lump in my throat and welling tears. I cleared my throat and pushed the tears away. "Can you please tell them?"

She agreed. The next day, the staff received the news. Later, I was told many of the nurses cried. One of their own had been struck down.

Chapter 8

EMOTIONAL TURBULENCE

Cancer is an experience of living life in extremes.

As a nurse, I had learned to keep my emotions in check and subdue them if needed to keep my head focused on my job. However, being diagnosed with cancer, my emotions took on their rawest form. Anger, sadness, fear, and tears swept over me at the strangest times. It was like being on a roller coaster ride...and I have never liked roller coasters.

"Please fill out this paperwork," the too-cheery receptionist at the outpatient cancer center said, handing me a clipboard and pen.

Sitting on the mauve-and rust-colored chair, I crossed my legs and wrote down answers to the questions. I felt calm in the brightly lit waiting area, which was accented with beige walls. I knew what was involved with a bone marrow biopsy, having assisted doctors with the procedure many times. I would receive a drug called Versed that would put me in a twilight sleep, and I'd forget the whole thing.

Skylar sat across from me, his elbows leaning on his knees, staring at the beige carpet.

I filled out general questions – name, age, address – and continued to more difficult questions: "Do you have cancer?

What kind of cancer? Date of diagnosis." My face felt as hot as a scorching fire, and I fumed with anger inside. *Are they kidding me? I actually have to answer this question?* The more I scribbled down answers, the more my anger raged. "This is making me so pissed off right now!"

"What?" Skylar asked, interrupted out of his fog.

"I actually have to write down on this paper that I have cancer. This is insane!" I exclaimed. "How can I have cancer?" I threw the pen down on the clipboard. "Here's another good one. Who is your oncologist? I can't believe I even have an oncologist!"

"This whole thing is pretty crazy," Skylar said, in a low, sad voice.

"Ugh." I gave him a look of frustration and picked up the pen, bit my tongue, and completed the questionnaire. I handed it to the receptionist and she escorted me to a patient room. Passing the circular nurses' station, I watched nurses working on their charts and heard the sound of an IV beeping. *How did I become the patient?*

I changed into a blue gown and lay on a hospital bed, listening to a jazz tune playing overhead. At least they tried to make this pleasant. The single-bed room looked white and sterile with a blue and maroon curtain hanging from the ceiling. A small window offered a view of a palm tree on the pretty July morning. In one corner stood a silver tray topped with clear-wrapped packages, the contents of one wrapped in blue Smurf tissue. I was used to seeing the needed equipment, but this time I couldn't believe it was for me. How strange.

A middle-aged nurse, wearing an old-school white uniform pants and top, came into the room. Her name badge hung around her neck on a lanyard made with pink ceramic beads. "Hi Christine, I'm Elise. I'm here to start your IV and assist in the procedure."

She attached a pulse oximeter to my finger. It read my oxygen saturation and heart rate. Then, she wrapped a blood pressure cuff on my arm that would take my pressure every five minutes during the procedure.

"Okay."

Elise sat in a chair next to my bed, donned a pair of gloves, and inserted a needle into my left hand. I silently critiqued her IV skills, which, fortunately, were good.

Dr. Mahdavi walked in wearing a lab coat and brown slacks. "Looks like you're relaxed and ready," he smiled, raising his thick salt-and-pepper mustache. "Any questions?"

I knew Dr. Mahdavi needed to do the biopsy to determine if the lymphoma had infiltrated my bone marrow. If so, I'd be diagnosed with stage four NHL, the worst.

"No, I know the deal," I said, surprisingly upbeat.

A long needle would be inserted into my lower back and a piece of bone marrow would be taken for testing. After the procedure, they'd apply a pressure bandage.

"Let me have you roll over onto your stomach," Elise said.

I complied.

"You're going to feel a little cold on your lower back," Dr. Mahdavi said. He scrubbed the procedure area with Betadine.

"Just try to rest, Christine," said Elise in a stiff tone, as she injected Versed into my IV.

The procedure was not traumatic. It was quick, and I didn't remember it at all which made me very happy.

After awakening in good spirits, I held Skylar's hand as we walked to the car, admiring the blue sky.

"They said you'll have a sore lower back tonight," he said, moving his sunglasses from his head to cover his eyes.

That was the least of my worries.

Days after my bone marrow biopsy, I shuffled down aisles in the small vitamin and health-food store, hearing the blades of a ceiling fan hum. I studied the assorted vitamin and herb jars as I searched frantically for something to help make me better. From one aisle to the other, assorted-sized jars tantalized customers with their claims to promote better health. The more I saw, the more confused I became.

I'd wakened encased in sweat. After quickly showering, I got dressed and drove to the store, my wet hair pulled up in a ponytail, feeling desperate. I picked up a soil brown-colored jar labeled "Skull Cap." The see-through bottle revealed beetle-sized tablets. I returned it to the shelf. *That can't be what I need.*

Over the last week, I'd started to come undone, feeling my life spiral out of control. I observed and felt my body going haywire, with more lumps in the back of my neck and under my armpits. New lumps seemed to appear daily. I felt disgusted. After undergoing weeks of tests, scheduling doctor appointments, and planning another surgery, a Port-a-Cath placement – a catheter inserted into a large chest vein – felt as if time was going in slow motion. Things weren't getting done fast enough, and I needed to do something to help myself. Nursing had taught me to assess the problem and then come up with an intervention. My intervention was to find something to boost my immune system.

I was overwhelmed. There were brown-bottled pills everywhere. I'd heard of some supplements, such as Echinacea, calcium, and magnesium, but I had no idea what many of the others were. I grabbed a brown dropper-sized jar, "milk thistle", and read the label. It made no sense and said nothing about the immune system, so I put it back on the shelf. I felt as if I was in a foreign country without any understanding of the language. I shuffled slowly down another aisle, examining the labels. Passing by jars of wormwood, COQ-10, cat's claw, and charcoal, my chest tightened in frustration. *Why is this so confusing?*

A thin Asian man with dark butterfly-wing eyebrows walked up. "Can I help you?"

"Uh, yes," I said as calmly as I could, even though I felt panicked. "I need to get something to help my immune system."

"Restore system?" he asked, in fragments with an Asian accent.

"Yes...that's exactly what I need." Wide-eyed, I grasped at his words.

He slowly and deliberately made his way to another aisle and handed me a blue box of tea entitled, "Immune Care."

"Helps function immune system, when not work," he said slowly.

"Oh, okay." I grabbed the box. "I'll take it."

One hour later, I sipped tea in a chair at my dining room table, my legs drawn up to my chest. I felt calmer and more in control, even if it did taste like watered-down dirt.

The sun barely peeked through the clouds as Skylar and I walked into Dr. Mahdavi's office a week later and sat in one of his patient rooms, waiting to hear my test results. I was scared, wondering how bad my diagnosis was. I tucked my fears within, ready to face facts. As an ER nurse, I was used to wearing a calm persona and containing my feelings.

I wrapped the large paper gown around my body to cover my backside, feeling like I was wearing a life-sized paper-doll cut-out. Skylar sat in a dark purple chair, and I stood in front of a framed, colored world map.

"Where do you want to go next?" I asked, displaying the world as if I was Vanna White.

"Ah, I don't know," Skylar said, in an uninterested tone, peering at his fashionable Cole Haan shoes.

"Well, I do." I pointed to the South Pacific. "I want to go to Tahiti, South America, and Italy."

Skylar smiled. "You're always my cheery girl, aren't ya?"

"Gotta have dreams and goals."

Dr. Mahdavi entered the room. I scurried to the exam table and sat down.

"Well, hello there," he said in a robust Santa Claus tone. "Looks like we're here to talk about some things."

I nodded. I lay back and Dr. Mahdavi examined my body, palpating under my arms, neck, groin area, and abdomen.

"I feel more lumps every day," I said. "It's so gross."

"Yes, I feel them. Let's talk about your test results." He crouched on a small stool. "The PET scan shows you have lymphoma throughout your lymph nodes, on both sides of your diaphragm." [7]

I glanced at Skylar. My heart raced, my senses suddenly heightened.

"The good news is the bone marrow biopsy is negative, so it's not stage four. You have stage three."

"Thank God," I said with relief, oddly focused on Dr. Mahdavi's off-white teeth and thin lips.

The doctor explained that he wanted me to have the chemo regimen of CHOP and Rituxan. The plan was to receive CHOP every three weeks, then Rituxan each second week after chemo. I would need at least six cycles, probably eight. [8]

I nodded to Dr. Mahdavi's words, pushing my fear aside. "I understand."

It seemed like our voices were amplified. There was a long pause in the room, and I shifted my body on the exam table, the tissue paper crackling underneath.

"You're probably not going to like this." I felt my face flush and guilt hung over me. I peered at the doctor's dark shiny shoes. "I started taking some tea to help boost my immune system."

"Stop taking the tea," he said calmly. "Why boost your immune system when it's defective?"

He was right. I'd never thought of that. I would stop drinking the tea. I logically knew this, but what my head and emotions said were two different things. I remembered some of my patients who had started holistic supplements and were later told by doctors not to. Doctors need to know about all medications prior to taking them. While many herbal supplements are good, some can have adverse interactions with cancer drugs. Before, I'd thought patients didn't trust the medical profession so they took matters into their own hands. But now I understood why. We all try to grasp at our minute straws of control amidst the cancer chaos.

Before the doctor left the room, Skylar shook Dr. Mahdavi's hand.

I got dressed and gave a deep sigh, feeling emotionally paralyzed.

"I made my decision," Skylar said.

"Decision for what?"

"I pick Africa. Let's go now."

Prior to receiving chemotherapy, a seemingly endless number of hospital procedures need to be performed: lab tests, an x-ray, and a Port-a-Cath, catheter-placement surgery. In some ways, it still didn't seem real and doubts about my diagnosis lingered in my mind. In the midst of this circus, I decided I wanted a second opinion.

While sitting in the back seat of my sister Karen's SUV, I gazed out at passing cars and gray pavement on our ride to the same hospital where I'd started my nursing career. I didn't say much to my mom and sister as they chatted in the front seat. Instead, I reminisced about my past work life on the surgical oncology floor and BMT unit.

I rested my arms on my stomach, closed my eyes, and nestled into the comfortable seat. I felt as if I were heading home, to a place filled with memories of myself at a simpler time. Among those memories, thoughts of a cancer patient for whom I'd cared came swirling into my head...

I entered room 214, pulled open the blue- and brown-checkered curtain, and detected the faint smell of disinfectant. My patient Ted, a sixty-three-year-old bald man, was lying in bed, a white sheet covering him from the waist down. He eyed me with curiosity through gold-framed glasses and interrupted his conversation with his wife, who sat in a chair across from him. A light blue hospital gown covered his thin body.

"Hi, my name's Christine and I'm your nurse for the day," I said enthusiastically.

A flicker of a smile brushed his mouth, and I saw a few of his yellow stained front teeth for an instant. Looking into his grayish blue eyes, I noticed despondency. I was hoping my upbeat attitude would make him feel somewhat better.

"I'm going to take your vital signs and do an assessment on you."

"Okay," he said, looking down at his freckled, weathered hands as they clasped the hem of the blanket.

While I performed my nursing duties, he began to talk. "My wife and I owned a dairy-farm business in Indiana. We just retired." Excitement filled his eyes.

"What brings you to hot California?" I asked.

"One of our dream trips was to come explore the sights in California. So here I am, with a hospital vacation and a diagnosis of cancer." His tone turned melancholy.

His wife sat in the chair and listened. Her oversized brown and white paisley dress formed the background for her yellow yarn and knitting needles. She was knitting a baby sweater. She looked like a woman who lived a country lifestyle; she wore her hair in a simple bun. Pulling her glasses to the bridge of her nose, she wiped a tear from under her eye.

After asking permission, I sat on his bed, feeling the softness of the brown woven blanket. I gave him my undivided attention. "I'm sorry you're going through this."

"Thanks," he said with a hint of a smile.

"Hopefully when you recover, you can see the California you came to see."

He looked deep into my eyes, interested in our conversation. In a bold voice, he said, "How old are you, young lady?"

"I'm twenty-four," I said shyly.

"Let me give you some advice. Don't wait until you retire to travel. We should have done this trip years ago, but the farm was just work, work, and work."

His words struck a chord in me. I knew these were words of wisdom flowing in the midst of his pain.

"It'll take some time to get through this, but don't give up on your dream yet," I said.

I gave him a hug. This practice of assisting my patients in the battlefield was making an impact on me. By witnessing the sadness and intensity of what they were living, I was developing a unique vantage point on life.

I walked over to Ted's wife, stooped down, and embraced her. With his words ringing in my mind, I felt complete assurance I would look at every moment of my life as an opportunity to live to the fullest.

It was then that I decided to become a world traveler.

"Well, it's good we're going to get a second opinion," Karen said, abruptly shaking me out of my reverie. The sun's warmth felt great on my bare arms. It also calmed me.

Karen stretched her head back to look at me. Her hazel eyes confirmed we were doing the right thing. She looked perfect: a clear complexion, straight brown hair, and straight teeth. As teenagers we fought a lot, but as adults we'd developed a nice friendship and support for each other. One of her lingering traits from high school was her tendency to reveal her concern by taking on a commanding tone of voice.

When Karen first saw me after surgery, she sat next to me on my futon couch at home and hysterically blurted, "Don't die on me!" She exploded into tears, questioning whether she'd been a good sister. I hugged her, realizing waves of shock and fear had overwhelmed her as well as me.

The July heat radiated off the black asphalt in the hospital parking lot. In one hand I gripped a poster-sized manila envelope, which read, "X-ray film, Please do not bend." I walked with my sister and Mom toward the scenic fountain at the hospital entrance. As we got closer, I heard the pleasant sound of water cascading into the round pool, but I felt anything but serene. My mind was confused, my thoughts bouncing from whether my diagnosis was mistaken to having the results confirmed so I could be confident moving forward. I begged for calm and order.

We walked into an exam room and waited for Dr. Prism, a lymphoma specialist. She and I had worked together on the BMT unit years earlier.

"This is such a great hospital. When you worked here, you always spoke so fondly of the staff and patients," my mom said, as she sat holding the envelope containing my PET scan, surgical report, and other related paperwork. Mom had a cushiony body and sea-blue eyes and always wore a genuine smile. No matter the situation, she remained upbeat, even though I could tell she was nervous.

"Uh huh," I said, once again sitting on a blue cushioned exam table in a cloth gown, tapping my feet nervously.

A moment later, Dr. Prism walked in wearing a purple chiffon blouse and camel-colored skirt, her name stitched in blue on her lab coat.

As she got closer, her face lit up into a smile. "It's great to see you. What are you doing here?" She gave me a strong hug.

A wave of comfort came over me, like seeing an old friend. "Well, you're not going to believe this," I said with hesitation. "I was diagnosed with stage three non-Hodgkin lymphoma." To her dumbfounded look, I said, "I know, what a weird twist."

Concerned, she pulled out the thick dark plastic PET scan, and pinned it up on the illuminated board. I told her about my surgery, and she read the other paperwork and then performed an exam.

"It's not that I don't trust my oncologist." I sounded apologetic. "I just want to make absolutely sure."

I stared up at her strong cheekbones while she palpated my lymph nodes. Strands of her red hair were tucked behind her ears. She wore white pearl earrings.

"Yes, you do have mixed-cell follicular non-Hodgkin lymphoma, stage three," she said with regret, then described the regimen of chemotherapy she would use. "You'll need standard treatment, CHOP, but I would give Rituxan on the same day as all the other chemo."

That was different. Dr. Mahdavi had wanted to give Rituxan the second week after chemo, and Dr. Prism said it wouldn't affect treatment adversely to give it on different days.

Dr. Prism sat on a stool in front of me. "Let me talk to all of you about the side effects of chemo," She looked at Mom and Karen, who stood near me by the exam table. "She'll lose her hair about three weeks after chemo starts and have potential side effects of nausea, constipation, mouth sores, and fatigue."

Karen and my mom nodded their heads. After discussing more symptoms and other things involved with treatment, she gave each of us a solid hug and a smile.

"She's a strong girl," Dr. Prism said as she left the room.

"I agree," Mom said loudly.

I felt reassured, like the weight of an elephant had fallen off me. For some reason, going back to the hospital where I had worked and receiving Dr. Prism's opinion made me feel more in control. Instead of feeling lost, I felt settled and more accepting of the path I needed to take.

The three of us walked out the front entrance. "Maybe you should drive up here for your treatment," Karen suggested.

"My insurance won't cover that. Besides, I trust and like Dr. Mahdavi."

Peace washed over me. I was soothed by the sun's warmth and glanced at the beautiful mountains in the near distance. Out of the corner of my eye, I watched a nurse wheel a thirty-something female patient to a car at the loading curb. The woman looked pale, with gaunt features, and wore a blue bandana covering her head. My heart grew heavy. I moved my eyes to the fountain next to me, and heard the pulse of cascading water. It was another reminder of how precious life's good times are. I said a prayer that her desperation would soon turn into hope.

Chapter 9

When Does It Begin?

Suffering causes the kind of vulnerability no one wants.

The cold outpatient surgery center was a stark contrast to the summer heat outside. I felt warm tucked inside a blanket, sitting on a gurney and wearing a surgical bonnet, ready for my Port-a-Cath (port) placement. The weeks of procedures, scans, and doctor's visits had felt like years. A port was the final thing I needed before beginning chemo. I was ready. This should be a piece of cake.

Dr. Kelsey's thick hand grabbed the rail of the metal gurney. His calming voice greeted me. "Ready for round two?"

"Sure, why not?" I said, in my most upbeat nurse voice. This surgery would be fast and easy. Working with ports for many years as an oncology nurse, I knew what to expect.[9]

The surgery lasted twenty minutes and was uneventful. An hour and a half later, I wore a bulky dressing on my upper left chest as I walked out of the surgery center, feeling fine.

While recuperating at Skylar's house, I watched him hover over the stove, cooking dinner. I leaned my back against a pillow, the armrest my support, and looked over the white-tiled bar and wooden barstools between us.

"I'm a little sore, but this was easier than my other surgery," I said, placing my hand on my V-necked teal t-shirt and feeling the dressing underneath.

"You deserve some easy days," he said, scooping hot pasta out of a metal pan. "We could make it a fun night and I could tip the gin bottle up to your port and pour." He laughed and tipped his cocktail toward me.

"Ha!" I grunted. "I'll stick with a pain pill for now." We ate dinner, watched television, and then headed to bed.

At 2:30 a.m., my eyes opened abruptly to sudden, strong pain. I tried to take a deep breath, but felt I couldn't expand my lungs fully. A gripping pain raged on the left side of my back. *Is someone stabbing me with a knife?*

I staggered out of bed and slowly made my way down the carpeted stairs, gripping the staircase railing, seized with fear. *What is happening?*

I sat in a wicker chair near the sliding glass door, hoping the pain would diminish.

The house was still except for the rhythm of a ticking clock. I stared out the window, noticing concrete slabs illuminated by the moon, keeping my breaths slow and shallow. I felt intense pain each time I attempted some deep breaths. I cried silently.

I heard the thump of Skylar's footsteps coming down the stairs. As his shadowed figure appeared, he cleared his throat. "What's going on?"

"It hurts ... to take a deep breath." I winced. "Feels like I'm being stabbed in the back with a knife."

He grew concerned. "Want me to take you to the hospital?"

"No, I can breathe." I paused. "It just hurts. I just need to sit up. I'll call the doctor in the morning."

I took a pain pill, and then sat in the chair for an hour, pondering my life. It was crumbling further. Eventually, I grew calmer, went back to bed, and slept until morning.

After calling Dr. Kelsey's office, I went to the hospital for a chest x-ray. An hour later, Skylar and I sat in Dr. Kelsey's office looking at the x-ray film of my white ribcage and shadowed lung fields against darkness.

"I'm so sorry," Dr. Kelsey said. "I slightly nicked your lung and gave you a pneumothorax." [10]

I paused and submerged my anger. *Great. Now I have one more thing to worry about!*

"Things are beginning to make sense," I replied, relieved to finally know what was going on. "I know it's a possibility with surgery."

"The good news is, it's so small that we don't need to put a chest tube in," he said. "It'll resolve on its own."

"Gotta look on the bright side," I said, hanging onto my happy persona. "Now I know how my patients feel."

I walked out of Dr. Kelsey's office, realizing each day would be different. I was in the war zone. The steep ups and downs of the roller coaster ride had begun.

Skylar and I drove south on Pacific Coast Highway after dropping off one of his kids at his ex-wife's house. I rested my head on the window and stared at the ocean, seeing evening clouds cover the sun. Introspective, I contemplated my changing life.

"Life is really strange. Don't you think?" I asked Skylar.

"Uh...yeah."

"I mean we were just having the time of our lives in Spain and Portugal and now I have cancer?"

"What's the saying, the only thing you can count on in life is change?"

Stopped at a traffic light, Skylar looked over his shoulder and made a turn into a beach parking lot.

"Where ya going?"

"Let's go watch the covered up sunset."

We exited the car and Skylar held my hand. In the distance the ocean looked more like winter than summer, with gray clouds filling the horizon. We sat on a bench.

I took a deep inhale, enjoying the smell of the ocean. The sound of the surf hitting the shore calmed me.

Skylar turned and looked at me. "The good thing about life is after the bad times hit the only way to go is up." He caressed my cheek, then stood and stuck his hand in his jeans pocket. He sat back down and placed a gold wedding band on my finger. "I hope you say yes and I hope this counts as one of those life-is-good moments."

My heart thumped with excitement. "Of course!" I embraced him and we kissed. "Yes!"

Skylar put his arm around my shoulder and we gazed at the ocean, resting in each other's happiness. A glimmer of hope had just arrived in the middle of my storm.

Later that month, Skylar and I drove to the cancer center. Shrubs highlighted the entrance to the two-story, off-white building, along with multi-colored tile benches. The entryway looked inviting, except for the words, "Cancer Center."

Before getting out of the car, I pulled down the visor, checking myself in the mirror. I looked like a healthy person and felt like one, except for the lumps, fatigue and night sweats. Despite how I looked or felt, the fact remained I was going in for my first round of chemotherapy.

We sat in the outdated chairs of Dr. Mahdavi's waiting room. My fingers were interlocked with Skylar's, our forearms resting on the wooden armrest. Touching shoulder to shoulder, I was comforted not only by his warmth, but by his calm demeanor and dependability. I scanned the small room. A rack full of magazines stared back, photos of glamorous movie stars with smiling faces, and their perfect bodies and expensive clothes plastered on the covers. A fake ficus tree stood in one corner looking pathetic, as though it'd been there for centuries. Two patients sat on either side of us.

The woman next to Skylar was puffy. She wore a lavender turban, had brown beady eyes and a cushingoid (moon) face, made round from steroids. She looked pale and ugly, and sighed frequently and deeply. She ended each sigh with "hmmm." The man sitting next to me was extremely underweight, with a hacking dry cough. He constantly clicked his fingernails on his black cane that rested on the chair. His wrinkles hung in striated layers and his head had sparse wisps of gray hair, reminding me of desert weeds. Both patients looked to be in their late sixties or seventies.

These people frightened me. *Am I in the Twilight Zone?* I nestled closer to Skylar for comfort. Putting my arms around his neck, I felt his stubble on my cheek and whispered, "I don't belong here." I rested my head on his shoulder, and sat silently.

"I know," he whispered.

I didn't belong to this group, nor did I ever want to.

I followed Nurse Rebecca into the chemo room, marching stiffly like a soldier, only looking where I needed to go. She escorted me to an aqua lounge chair, with Skylar following. I was nervous, and already irritated from the coldness in the room. I put on a fluffy sweater. I held a book and portable CD player. I'd tried to plan accordingly; they told me I'd be there at least three hours. I figured I would use music, reading, and deep breathing to shut out my surroundings and help get me through it.

Skylar plopped down in a plastic cafeteria-type chair next to me. "Ya okay?"

I nodded. My attention was drawn to Nurse Rebecca, who dragged a wheeled, portable metal tray over the brown carpet. It carried sterile-packaged items needed to access my Port-a-Cath. Nurse Rebecca wore her platinum blond hair short, the sides of her hair only about a half-inch thick. It reminded me of a military cut. Her eyes were decorated with dark make-up. She looked to be in her mid-forties, had a curvy figure, and seemed to have an edge about her.

"Okay, Christine, I'm going to access your port and give you some Kytril [anti-nausea medication]," she said with a huff, appearing annoyed with me already. *Really?* I wondered if I looked the same way when I was busy with my patients.

She must have sensed I was guarded, wanting to keep the others out, including her. "Yeah. Okay. Do it."

She donned her gloves for the sterile procedure. I felt the coolness of the Betadine swab, and then got a whiff of alcohol as she rubbed the swab sticks on my port and around the area. I tensed, thinking how this was something I smelled every day and never thought anything of it. Now, I loathed it.

She took a quarter-inch needle, and pushed it into my port. I felt resistance, like a pushpin through a bulletin board, a reminder that something foreign was in my body. She withdrew a little blood with a syringe, making sure the needle was in place.

"You can leave," I said, squeezing Skylar's hand. "I'll be okay." I knew he wanted to be by my side. *No one wants to be here, so why should he?*

"She's most likely gonna be tired from the treatment anyway," Rebecca said, her hair rubbing the neckline of her polka-dot scrub top. She started an IV infusion.

Skylar kissed my forehead and left. A nurse would call him when I was close to being done.

Nestling back in the lounge chair, I heard the clicking of the IV pump. The medical equipment and healthcare environment was second nature to me. Now, though, it stressed me; I wanted to protect myself from it. I closed my eyes and took some deep breaths.

Fifteen minutes later, Nurse Rebecca said, "I have your chemo here." I opened my eyes and saw her Smurf-gloved hands inject a clear fluid-filled syringe into my IV line.

I needed to relax, so I put my ear buds in and listened to yoga-type music. I fidgeted in my seat and then scanned the room.

The eggshell-colored space was half the size of a tennis court. Windows ran three-fourths the way up one wall, allowing natural light in and a small blue-sky view. There were six recliner chairs as well as a stand-up scale, three metal hip-high trays, and a portable vital sign machine.

Three elderly patients were reclining in their chairs, relaxed. I glanced at the one across from me who wore a beige fishing hat over her head. She smiled at me wanly, accentuating her hollow cancer features. Bothered, I didn't smile back. I gazed at my CD player and closed my eyes, wanting to maintain my protective barrier.

Rebecca spiked the IV tubing into a chemo bag and then hung the Kool-Aid-red bag onto the IV pole. I could smell the remnants of chemicals, confirmation that I was being pumped full of poison. Anger raged inside me. I didn't want to look at any of it – the patients, the IV bag, or the room.

An hour later, I walked to the bathroom, wheeling my IV pole awkwardly in tow. The tubing connected me and this metal coat rack on which I had to depend. As I urinated, the harsh, disgusting odor of the chemicals rose up to my nose. When I flushed the toilet, I saw the Kool-Aid red color in the bowl. The assault on my body left me sickened, fearful.

I was in a haze during the twenty-five minute drive home. I rested my head on the passenger's side window of Skylar's car, drugged and out of it. All I wanted to do was get home and collapse into bed.

Skylar's car motored toward what was now our home. I moved in with him before my treatment began, and put my condo up for sale. Getting engaged had cemented our relationship further. The car air conditioner blew cool air, a small comfort that helped me fall asleep.

I roused when Skylar rounded a corner two streets before the house. A sick, gurgly feeling lurked in my stomach. It crept up to my throat. I attempted to submerge the queasy feeling by looking at the houses moving past, but couldn't. I grabbed onto the door handle and stared at the gray car interior, trying to make my insides stay still. While strangling the handle, I shimmied with the movement of another turn.

"How're you feeling?" Skylar asked.

I couldn't respond. Nausea and the fear of throwing up were inching closer.

Another turn sloshed my stomach's contents from side to side. I burped, tasting acid. I pushed it down by swallowing frequently.

Skylar stopped in our driveway. I flung the car door open, my right foot slamming onto the concrete driveway, my left foot on the grass. It hit me fast and powerfully. I crumbled to all fours, puking violently onto the grass. The depths of my intestines landed on the blades of grass, as if a fastball had been thrown out of me. My stomach convulsed, ejecting thick sputum and gold-colored vomit. The noise coming from me was agonizing, like a mother giving birth. My hands clawed at the grass, trying to hold onto anything solid. I felt as if I were on a teeter-totter. Tears erupted from my eyes. I was helpless, utterly out of control.

The angled brown shutters blocked most of the afternoon sunlight as it tried to stream into the living room. I'd found respite on the beige woven couch. I rested my head on a light-blue pillow, curled up in a ball, feeling the awful effects of chemo screeching through my body. All I could do was close my eyes, lie there, and take the agony.

The clunk of a glass tumbler on the coffee table made me open my eyelids.

"Honey, try to drink some water," Skylar said. "You need to drink so you don't get dehydrated." His palm brushed the top of my head, smoothing out my hair. I fell back asleep.

I was startled back to consciousness by a return of the nausea. It swept through my whole being. I couldn't focus on anything else but the horrid monster inside me. As my stomach sloshed, thick saliva coated my mouth and sourness lodged in the back edges of my throat. I'd had gastrointestinal flus, but this was worse ... the sickest I'd ever felt.

The grotesque feeling got worse. Rage churned inside me. "Oh, God," I yelled, and ran into the bathroom, trying to hold it back. Shoving the bathroom door open with one hand, and covering my mouth with the other, I struggled to reach the toilet.

I couldn't hold it in. Watery yellow vomit spewed onto the bathroom floor. I frantically crouched at the toilet, holding onto the sides of it as my body quivered. In a strong wave, more vomit dumped into the toilet. My stomach convulsed again, expelling more, loudly and violently. Hoping for a break, I crossed my arms on top of the toilet seat, and rested my head. I stared at the thread of thick saliva escaping my mouth, coiling into the water.

With the back of my hand, I rubbed tears from my eyes and spit saliva remnants into the toilet.

Skylar tapped on the partially opened door and said, "Honey, are you okay?"

"Yeah," I said, my voice echoing, embarrassment gripping me. I barely lifted my head off the toilet seat. "Please leave me alone."

He walked away.

I took a royal blue towel from the rack and wiped my face, blew my nose with a tissue, then sat on the cool ceramic floor depleted. I realized I could only get through this minute by minute.

An hour later, I opened my eyes after a nap. I blinked, focusing on glass knickknacks and a Lladro statue in the wooden hutch. A pile of tennis shoes were stacked on the floor next to it. The living room light had changed to a late-day orange; it was 6:00 p.m. On the coffee table was a glass filled with water and a green plastic Tupperware bowl. Not wanting to move from my horizontal position on the couch, I assessed how I felt.

In the kitchen, Skylar was sorting through the mail, glasses on his nose. "How ya doing?" he asked in a low voice. Tilting his nose down, he peered above his glasses. "I put a bucket there just in case it's too hard to get to the bathroom."

"Thanks." I rested my head on the pillow. "I'm still nauseous." I felt a thick paste on my tongue and took a sip of water. "I'd better take a Zofran [anti-nausea medication]."

Four pill bottles were lined up on the bar. I took out a foil-wrapped Zofran, slipped my fingernail between the folds of the pouch, and emptied a round, chalky pill into my palm. I'd never had the type of Zofran taken under the tongue (sublingual) before; in the hospital, I'd given it to patients via IV or orally. After popping it under my tongue, I tasted a sickening combination of paste and buttermilk. I gagged from the sourness.

"It's horrible." I grabbed the glass of water and took some sips. "I need some crackers."

Skylar dashed to the pantry. He handed me some saltines and I took a bite. I chewed carefully, worried I would puke. After swallowing, I held my bucket in front of me as if it were a tub of popcorn.

"I feel so sick," I said sadly. "This nausea is horrid. I think it's worse than throwing up." I shook my head, attempting to rid myself of the *I'm-going-to-die* feeling. "At least with the flu you usually have a little time to make it to the bathroom. Not with this." I took another sip of water, making a pouty face. "Yuck. Even water doesn't seem right. Everything tastes like a mixture of metal and cardboard." I remembered some of my patients' telling me food didn't taste the same.

I curled my legs up to my chest and held them close, and put my head down on the pillow, trying to think of other things.

An hour later, I was still nauseous. "This stuff doesn't work," I said, frustrated.

I grabbed a glass of Gatorade, took a Compazine, another anti-nausea pill, and again laid my head on the pillow. I contemplated how to muster up the courage to take another pill.

Half an hour later, Skylar made me some toast. I needed to take the prednisone with food. [11]

Like a fearful child, I held the Tic-Tac-sized round prednisone pill in the palm of my hand, trying to convince myself how small it was and that it wasn't a big deal to swallow it. I gulped some Gatorade and popped the pill into my mouth. *Bitter.* "Yuck. That's gross, too." I couldn't believe swallowing a pill was so difficult.

I grabbed my bucket and again placed it in my lap, an uneasiness lurking in my stomach. Rubbing the thick edges of the Tupperware bowl with my fingers, my mind drifted to memories of many oncology patients I'd cared for over the years. I'd stood at their bedsides, waiting patiently for them to take their pills, and noticing how difficult it was for them.

Now I knew their misery. Now I understood why this simple task proved to be a hardship.

By 8:00 p.m., twilight was inching its way into darkness. Exhausted, I wanted the comfort of lying down in bed. Slowly I climbed the carpeted stairs, holding onto the wooden railing. I stopped to rest on one of the stairs, amazed at how worn out I was. I'd only had one chemo treatment, and I couldn't even walk up a flight of stairs. Ugh. I grabbed the rail tightly and pulled myself up four steps, then rested. Unbelievable. I used to do spin classes and hike around Europe. Now, I couldn't even climb to my bedroom. I continued my ascent, stopping one more time before making it to the top.

When I finally reached the bed, I lifted the cotton green sheet up over my shoulders. I'd thrown up six times on this first day. My body was in hell. I closed my eyes. My lesson from day one: Sleep is my new best friend.

Three days later, I trudged into the chemo room, trailing Nurse Rebecca to a recliner. Plopping my fatigued body in a chair, I held a gold-colored emesis basin, the ugliness of nausea lurking. Dark circles were etched below my eyes, highlighting the dimness in my body and soul. My healthy glow was gone, replaced with a window into the revolt being waged inside. I teetered on the ledge of misery. I wanted so much just to feel a little bit better.

The previous two days had been filled with nausea; I threw up at least five times each day. My days consisted of nausea, sleep, taking pills, nausea, and struggling to eat and drink. I'd been prescribed Ativan, another medication for nausea. It helped for a while, but the queasiness kept coming back. I called the doctor's office, notifying them that I was barely able to keep fluids or food down. They wanted me to come in for a hydration IV and more medication.

I sat in the recliner, listless and depleted, knowing I couldn't do what I needed to do.

"Nothing stays down for long," I told Nurse Rebecca, while she accessed my port. "I can't drink much water."

She hung an IV fluid of saline, dextrose, and potassium and gave me IV anti-nausea medication. "It's not easy, but you've gotta drink more fluids," she said with a motherly look. "You're dehydrated." She handed me a glass of water.

"I get it." I sipped the water as if it were mouthwash.

I was an oncology nurse for years! Why am I not doing better with this? Why is this happening to me?

I had no idea chemo would be this terrible. The poison that was pumped into my system had to be working. The weeds in my immune system–the cancer cells in my lymph nodes – were hopefully shriveling and dying in combat. [12]

I opened my eyes and looked up at the plastic IV bag hanging on the metal pole. It was three-quarters empty. I repositioned myself to sit more upright in the chair and noticed the room was bright with natural light. It was 11:00 a.m., two hours after I'd arrived feeling half dead. Now feeling better, I became aware of other patients chatting. A wave of embarrassment set in when I realized they all had seen my misery. I was barely surviving. I ignored them, covering myself with a brown sweater and closing my eyes.

Half an hour later, I walked out of the chemo room and into the waiting room. Skylar looked handsome as he waited on a side chair.

"I feel so much better," I said, giving him a hug and a bright smile.

"Now you're back to my perky girl again."

He held me close. I was comforted in his embrace, thankful for his warmth and love.

Like a wilted flower just watered, my petals lifted back to life. Even the dark bags under my eyes had returned to normal. I felt energetic, my soul re-integrated into myself. *Thank you, God.* We walked out of the cancer center, arm in arm. Looking beyond a color-tiled bench, I saw a pink hydrangea. I smiled. It's amazing what water can do.

Chapter 10

Life on the Other Side

I headed into the chemo room on a hot August afternoon, wearing a knee-length white denim skirt and turquoise tank top. The air conditioner roared up an arctic winter blast. I slipped my thick cream-colored sweater on, melting into its cashmere softness.

For more reasons than the weather, I wanted to be outside. I was feeling like myself again, eating and drinking well. I followed Nurse Rebecca to a chair in the chemo room, knowing where I belonged, yet filled with resistance and uneasiness about my Rituxan treatment. I heard the conversation of other patients, even laughter, and thought, *this isn't a place to act like everything is okay*. I just wanted to be quiet, get through it, and move on. I shut out their happiness.

Nurse Rebecca took my vital signs and accessed my port.

"I'm gonna give you some Benadryl as a pre-med before the Rituxan." Her tone was matter-of-fact, her guard up, which I was starting to understand more and even liked. Maybe she and I had both learned we needed to have certain boundaries to be able to work in a field where there's so much sadness. "You'll probably be drowsy in a bit here, so it would be better to chat now."

You gotta be kidding me. Why? I gave her a thin, half-sincere smile and fiddled with my CD player.

Two other patients were in the room. The woman looked to be in her late fifties. She wore a powder-blue bandana, shimmery white eyeshadow, and thick brown eyeliner. She was wearing nighttime eye make-up, but whatever.

The other patient was a man in his seventies. He wore a blue and white Hawaiian shirt and khaki shorts, covering his thick robust body. He had dull blue eyes and sported a bronze tan. He reminded me of a salty sailor, someone who'd worked on boats his whole life.

"How ya doing today?" he asked in a deep voice.

I glanced at him and then at the eyeshadow lady. She looked straight at me and smiled.

"Uh, I'm okay." I was put off by his verbal intrusion.

"So what's wrong with you?" He spilled another intrusive question.

"Uh, I have non-Hodgkin lymphoma," I said, thinking he'd probably never heard of it.

A smile crossed his face. "That's what I have."

"Really?"

"Yeah, this is my fourth Rituxan treatment. I'm also getting CHOP chemo."

"That's what I'm getting," I said, surprised and relieved, letting my guard slip.

"Okay, Christine, I'm starting your Rituxan now," Nurse Rebecca said. [13]

"This is my first Rituxan treatment," I said. "I had my first CHOP treatment. It was brutal. I threw up a lot."

"That's too bad." He tapped his thumb on the side of the chair. "I've been really fortunate. I've hardly had any side effects. That day I get a little nausea, but that's it."

Lucky guy. I looked down at my antsy legs. I stuck them straight out, then moved my feet up and down as if I were a ballerina doing toe exercises. I tapped them on the rug to help get rid of the pins-and-needles feeling.

"Benadryl makes my legs feel weird," I said.

"It's funny how all this stuff affects people differently."

Yeah.

Eyeshadow lady spoke up. "How old are you, Honey?"

"Thirty-eight," I said, in a light-hearted tone, "and I've been an oncology nurse."

An uncomfortable silence filled the room. Then the Hawaiian-shirt guy said, "Well, now you're in the club."

"The club?"

"Yeah, we're all in the club, a club we never wanted to be in, but here we are."

I stretched my lips to a half-smile and shut my eyes. Though feeling uncomfortable amongst "them," the fact remained; I was now one of them.

It had been two and a half weeks since my first chemo, and my energy level and appetite were back. For that, I was thankful.

While sitting in a booth at a Marie Callendar's restaurant, I listened to overhead music, the clatter of silverware, and the murmur of conversations. I sat with shoulders touching the mahogany wooden seat back, my posture perfect. Across from me were my mom and her best friend, Lois. They took me to lunch, to see how I was doing.

My stomach grumbled. I eyed the poster-sized menu, trying to figure out what I wanted. After taking the Rituxan, I felt tired the rest of the day, but after that I was fine. I looked forward to a satisfying lunch, and tried to ignore the gnawing anger inside of me.

"I'm gonna get a burger," I said, feeling my curly hair brush my cheeks.

I gazed at my mom and Lois. Lois had been our next-door neighbor, "my other mother," since I was five years old. She'd taught me how to bake Texas sheet cake. Now, she was a seventy-year-old, red-haired smoker.

"I like your hair short like that. It's a pixie cut," Lois said in her deep smoker's voice.

"I don't like it," I pouted. "I cut it shorter so I wouldn't shed long strands of hair all over the place and make a mess. It's coming out more now."

"At least you have your appetite back," my mom said with a hearty smile.

"Wow, big deal, I get to eat like a normal person." My volume rose.

They lifted their eyebrows and looked at each other, surprised at my sour attitude. Very uncharacteristic.

The sparks of my anger rubbed together like flint, igniting more irritation. "I just want to know why this is happening to me."

Mom's eyes pierced mine. "What did the doctors say?"

"They say they don't know what caused it." I looked down at the forest-green napkin in my lap. "Why doesn't anyone know?" I lifted my hands, spreading my fingers out as if I was wearing a baseball mitt, expecting to catch the answer in my palm. "It makes no sense. I didn't do anything to deserve this."

"You're right," my mom said, sadness in her voice. "None of this makes sense."

Tension tightened my neck and jaw. "It's not fair!"

"You absolutely have a right to be upset," Lois said, leaning her skinny elbows onto the table. "But I'm worried about you. I've never seen you this angry."

"Oh yeah, well I'm pissed off!" My face turned red, and I clenched my fists in my lap. "I feel like taking an ice pick and destroying this bench." I beheld my serrated knife resting on the table. My pulse raced, fury boiling inside.

A plump, young waitress with shiny black hair came to the table. "Ready to order?"

They ordered first. I took a deep breath, feeling the heat diminish in my face. "I'll have a cheeseburger and fries," I said, snapping back into a calmer tone.

Silence filled the table as we regrouped.

"You've been dealt a hand no one would want," my mom said. "It's understandable why you're angry about it."

"This whole thing makes no sense," I repeated, begging for an answer.

"I absolutely agree. I think you've gotta put these questions aside and just try to focus on getting better."

That irritated me more. "Of course I'm focused on getting better." I rolled my eyes. "Don't worry, I'm not going to destroy anything," I said, feeling I needed to defend myself, ensuring them I wasn't going to go berserk.

Ten minutes passed, and the waitress came with our food. I took a sip of lemonade.

"Maybe it would help to think more positively," Mom said.

I shot a piercing glare at her. "Are you kidding me, think positive?" I shouted. People in neighboring booths started to stare. "What the hell is there to think positive about? I have to go back in two days and have the same thing happen all over again." I glanced down at my napkin. Not wanting to alienate my support team, I subdued myself. "I can't talk about this anymore."

The red, hot lava of my rage spewed inside. *That's the worst advice I've ever heard. If I could think positive, I would.*

I ate my burger. I knew what people shouldn't say. Sometimes, it's better for loved ones to just listen.

The house was quiet. I was alone wandering from room to room, feeling out of sorts. Skylar was at work. It was the fifth day after my second round of chemo and, like the first, I had been sick as a dog, puking for four days and unable to keep food down or drink many fluids. I'd gone to the cancer center for another hydration IV. Now, one day later, I needed to lie down. Instead of lying in our bed or on the couch, I needed a change of scenery.

I walked into the guest bedroom, seeing the morning sun shine through the slats of the closed wooden shutters. I didn't want to see the beauty of the summer day. I wanted to shut out the reminders of the active person I used to be. Now I spent all my days doing nothing but either lying on the couch or getting treatments. My double bed and white-washed desk were amidst a shelf of trophies, a pile of clean clothes, and baseball paraphernalia. We used the room as an extra bedroom for Skylar's kids when they came for a weekend. I grabbed my spiral-bound journal and plopped on the bed. Depressed, I pet the green woven blanket, pondering my losses. I opened the green and white daisy-covered journal, and peered inside the cover. Cassie, an ER tech, had given it to me. She had written, "Store your thoughts and feelings in this journal and ease your mind." I rubbed my hand on the sweetly decorated page. Assorted stickers of hearts, flowers, a butterfly, and a dog filled the page, along with the words "faith," "friends," and "be happy."

That morning I'd rinsed my hair after shampooing and found a clump in my hand. I stared at the tangled glob as water cascaded over it. Even though I knew it was going to happen, it was still a surprise. I rubbed it off and watched it whisk down the drain. My life had changed dramatically.

Living in my condo, working, and traveling were things of the past. I wasn't happy about letting go of my old self. I liked living a fun, fast-paced life. Now, I lived at a snail's pace. Clump by clump, remnants of my old life were being shed. Stripped of the person I used to be, I needed encouragement and a release. Badly.

I grabbed a Bible from the desk shelf and opened it, hoping the words would grab me. I flipped through the thin pages, and read segments but had trouble concentrating on the words. My mind was dazed. I put it aside. Gripping the journal, I lay sideways on the bed with my head on my arm and began writing. *Maybe, instead of taking things in, I needed to get them out.*

I felt some relief from the swirls of letters I wrote on the page. "This is a difficult process!" I wrote. "It is filled with emotional self-reflection, a time of watching my body do things I never dreamed or imagined it would do."

My anger and depression escaped onto the page, giving me relief. It was hard coping with my illness and maneuvering through this trial. Little by little, whether journaling, talking to Skylar, or punching the Bozo the Clown punching bag Mom bought me soon after our Marie Callendar's lunch episode, I needed to experience every feeling and get them out. No matter how horrible.

I continued writing. Maybe someday I could piece the trauma and craziness together. "Being a cancer patient takes a lot of courage."

Days later, I sat shoulder to shoulder with Skylar on the couch, staring at the television screen, mesmerized by the green grass of the baseball diamond.

"Did you hear what I said?" Skylar asked.

He was immaculately dressed in a white polo shirt and Bermuda shorts. As he took sips from a Heineken, a baseball announcer bellowed from the television.

"Uh, no," I said, moving my gaze from the television to him, shaking myself out of a daze. "What did you say?"

I removed my feet from the coffee table and placed one leg on the couch, facing him.

He scratched the bristles of his silver-and sand-colored beard. "Remember I told you yesterday the kids are coming over later?"

I noticed a hint of irritation.

"You didn't tell me that." I felt sure of my memory-recall capabilities.

"Honey, yes I did."

"Oh. Okay." I was a little embarrassed. "I guess chemo brain has set in." It *had* been getting worse.[14]

"Either that or you're becoming ditzy," he chuckled.

"Thanks a lot." I lightly slugged his arm. "Wanna play Rack-o?"

Rack-o is a simple card game in which players arrange cards in numerical order. It would help me concentrate on something so I wouldn't focus on how I was feeling, usually nauseated or down.

"Sure."

I pulled the box from under the glass-topped coffee table and set up the cards and plastic racks between us on the couch. Skylar dealt the cards.

"Who woulda thought a kid's game would be so comforting?" I rubbed the edge of a card's stiffness between my fingertips and placed it into a rack. I focused on putting cards in numerical order. All I could focus on. I took a deep breath and pondered how sad and ironic that my life was anything but orderly these days.

Friday night, a coastal fog had drawn onto land. It reminded me of fall, giving me a teaser of time passing, something I desperately wanted.

Wearing white shorts and a fuchsia-colored t-shirt, I briskly walked the kitchen and family room, attempting to rid myself of the bloating, heaviness, and discomfort I felt. On Friday nights in the past, I would have been out with friends or Skylar, or working. Now, I felt awful, dealing with constipation for the last three days due to the chemotherapy Vincristine. *Is there anything resembling normal in this process?*

"I feel gross," I told Skylar as I walked with a determined gait into the kitchen from the family room, my third lap. "I have cramping pains." I'd been drinking lots of water and prune juice, and even took a Dulcolax tablet, hoping for quick results.

I turned around in the kitchen, and headed to the family room, where I heard dialogue from some television show.

"It's gotta come out sooner or later," Skylar said, sitting on a barstool in the kitchen, gripping a small glass tumbler full of a vodka-cranberry cocktail.

With a quick stride, I pumped my arms, fierce with the movement of a power-walker.

Skylar raised his glass. "You go, girl!" He smiled, cheering as if he were a spectator at a marathon.

"Our Friday night excitement. Woo hoo!" I took one more lap from the family room into the kitchen. "I gotta rest."

I sat down at the round glass table I'd once had in my condo, and heard the wicker chair creak. I picked up a paintbrush and continued where I'd left off with my paint-by-number. I'd reverted to simple things for entertainment, a detour from whatever internal discomfort was going on. I guess it's comforting to slip back to simpler times in life.

An hour passed. "Here goes..." I headed to the bathroom.

Afterwards, I walked back into the kitchen. Skylar was sipping his third cocktail. I jumped up and down on the white-tiled floor yelling, "Yay! I feel so much better." I ran to him, and we high-fived.

"See, it was a rip-roaring Friday night after all," he laughed.

Rubbing my belly and feeling lighter, I thought, *It's amazing how big small victories can be.*

Chapter 11

REMOVING BITS OF MYSELF

My morning entertainment was watching sparrows flitter in and out of a backyard bush as I was sitting on the couch, looking through the sliding glass door, the television occupying the other half of my attention. I didn't know what to do with myself, a non-working woman on disability. I tucked my legs under me, put my elbow on the armrest, and stared blankly at the mute screen, dazed.

I scratched my scalp. It was tender. I gently moved my fingers to different areas of my head; it all felt sore. I combed my fingers through my hair, displeased by its coarse sandpaper texture.

"Gross," I said aloud. A brown clump of hair sat on the edge of my fingertips, looking like a matted fur-ball. It scared me to see it. I rubbed it ... it was sticky. "That's it," I said, irritated.

My hair had to come off. As I held this changed piece of myself, I remembered a patient of mine named Edward on the BMT unit. Maybe I hadn't really understood the meaning of shaving a person's head.

I had stood in the anteroom next to Edward's room on the BMT unit, wearing a yellow gown, blue booties, a blue surgical cap, and a mask. The required gear made me hot, but it was standard protocol for the critical time after a patient receives a bone marrow transplant. I walked swiftly into his isolation room, a portable electric shaver in my hand. He'd already received high-dose chemotherapy and radiation to obliterate his defective white blood cells caused by leukemia.

"Hi Edward. Ya ready for this?"

Edward was twenty-seven years old with brown skin, chubby cheeks, and a shy smile. He loved playing soccer and worked as an auto mechanic before cancer struck him down. A poster of the soccer icon, Pele, hung in his room.

I put towels on the floor around a chair, and prepped the area for shaving his head. I peered over my shoulder, and saw him lying in bed, his brown eyes tired. He carefully held onto the beige side rail, and lifted himself off the bed, his pillow covered with short black hairs. IV tubes were connected to four IV pumps and dangled from his chest like jump ropes. He moved to the "barber's chair," and sat with his head tilted down, hands clasped together.

"Are ya okay?" He nodded. He'd developed mouth sores from the chemo, so I understood he probably didn't want to talk. "Is it okay if I start shaving?"

He nodded again and scratched his head.

I moved behind him and patted his shoulder. The room's backlighting cast a butterscotch glow. Only the size of a large closet, the room contained a single bed, bedside table, nurse's pantry, sofa-type chair, smaller chair, and bathroom.

The shaver buzzed and vibrated in my hand. With each pass, pieces of his hair lifted into its metal teeth. Clumps fell onto the towel covering his shoulders. Black hair covered the floor.

Five minutes later, I announced, "All done."

He took his hands and rubbed his head. Razor-sized bits of hair fell.

"How does it feel?"

"Pretty good," he said in a low voice.

I disconnected him from his IVs so he could take a shower. While I cleaned up the towels and hair on the floor, my mind turned to other tasks of the day.

The moment when a chemo patient begins to lose his or her hair is often very traumatic. For many, when it begins to fall out in large, ugly clumps, it's time to shave it off. Many cannot bear to watch their hair fall out slowly and randomly. Shaving it offers a feeling of control over the situation. I had helped a number of patients like Edward at this difficult time.

Now, I knew how it felt.

I picked up the portable phone and called my sister. "My hair feels disgusting," I said, resolve in my tone. "It's time to shave it off."

"Ah, okay. We figured that was coming."

Karen lived in the same town as my parents, whom I was planning to visit for the weekend. She'd bought me silk floral scarves and a checkered blue and white bandana when we'd gone shopping the week before.

"Okay, I'll tell Andy to get the shaver ready for tomorrow," she said.

Andy, my brother-in-law, regularly shaved his head. A six-foot-tall, thirty-something surfer, he'd been married to my sister for years. They had two daughters, ages seven and three.

I hung up the phone and walked to the kitchen, throwing the hairball away. Another thing I needed to let go of.

A few days later, I lay exhausted on a feather pillow on the striped living room couch at my parents' house, an hour inland from where I lived. With my energy sapped from the drive and the heat, I was thankful for the coolness from the air-conditioner, which helped me relax. My mom watched me from her over-sized aqua chair. I heard muted conversation between my brother-in-law and sister, and knew they were setting up the kitchen to shave my head. I dozed off, glad I was with my family.

Sometime later, I was roused by the excited shrills of my two nieces, running towards me. "Auntie, we have a picture for you."

With exuberant faces and bouncing blonde hair, they rushed into my arms and thrust crayon pictures at me.

"That is so sweet – thank you!" I embraced them and inhaled the fresh berry scent of their shampoo.

I lifted my head from the pillow, and noticed brown, curly hairs covering it. I looked away.

"Auntie, you have to get rid of your hair today?" the seven-year-old asked.

"Yeah, but it's okay. Wanna see what my head looks like without hair?"

"Okay," they replied in unison.

We headed to the kitchen, passing my dad in the family room. He had a crooked nose and wore a white t-shirt that showed his farmer's tan. Known for his offbeat sense of humor, Dad also dealt with his share of difficult medical issues. My first year out of high school, he was involved in a devastating head-on collision. The doctors doubted he would live. Then they told us it was unlikely he would ever walk again. He did, and even returned to his job as a construction worker.

"Ready to go for the chrome-dome look?" my dad asked me.

"Yeah, gotta get it shaved. It's time." I shrugged my shoulders.

Thankful for my family cheerleaders, I headed into the kitchen, throwing away a handful of hair in the trash. A canary-colored sheet lay on the linoleum floor, a wooden chair in the middle of it. The kitchen's yellow walls and many windows made it an energetic place to be.

I sat down, and Andy grabbed the shaver. My mom, nieces, and sister stood in the kitchen, watching.

I tipped my head down. I heard the buzz of the razor and felt the vibration on my scalp. Strips of hair fell onto the sheet. I twinged with grief, but then glanced up at my nieces, their eyes wide. They made me smile.

I peered down at the floor as more hair cascaded to the ground. Compared to other things I needed to endure, it wasn't that bad.

Five minutes later, Andy announced, "You're done."

I rubbed my scalp with my hands, and smiled. "It feels kinda weird. I feel lighter."

"You look good," my mom said in an exuberant tone.

"You have a really good head," my sister said.

I knew what she meant. Some of my patients had lumps on their heads.

"Yah, Auntie," the three-year-old said.

After removing the towels covering my shoulders, I brushed leftover hair off my body. "Wanna feel my head?" I asked my nieces.

They ran toward me. I bent to the ground and felt their cool hands rub my scalp. "It feels really soft," the seven-year-old said.

I patted my head. "Yeah, you're right."

I walked to a mirror in the entryway. "This is different," I said, peering at my mannequin-like head, trying to get used to my changed reflection in the mirror. "I guess now I'll experience life as a bald woman."

An hour later, I was coloring in a coloring book with my nieces, feeling content. I was changing. Not only were there many physical issues to deal with, but I was also learning to depend on others for help, instead of trying to be Miss Independent. Not easy, but I had to let go and allow others to assist me. No way I could do the cancer experience alone.

Chapter 12

PERCEPTIONS

This is a difficult process filled with emotional self-reflection. It's a time of watching my body do things I never imagined or dreamed it would do.

It was a long, hot beginning of September night. Four pillows cushioned my bald head. I had woken up abruptly, propped myself upright, and stared into the dark bedroom. Crickets chirped, and the ceiling fan hummed. Worry began to consume me. How would I psych myself up for my third chemo treatment tomorrow? My mind darted with thoughts, one crazy, one rational, churning my stomach along with it. *Why isn't Skylar next to me? Does he find me unattractive and want to leave me?*

Our times of intimacy had dwindled. Understandable. As I looked at the dresser, wreathed in shadow and topped with a television, I pondered how to calm my anxious mind. *You're okay. Simmer down.* I rubbed the cotton sheet between my fingers and drew my eyes up to the closed blinds. How could I walk into the chemo room knowing what hell is coming?

My heart raced. I ruminated about the suffering that lurked ahead. I closed my eyes and tried to pray, but couldn't.

Instead, worry plagued my mind. My thoughts spiraled into a dark hole. *Sometimes I can barely walk up the stairs.*

How could I get through this next round? Would I ever again be the woman I was? Why did my life have to change? *I don't even know who this worrying person is. This isn't me. I am a functional, productive person.*

I touched my port, a hard lump that stuck out conspicuously when I wore lower-necked tops. As a result, some of my favorite clothes were relegated to the back of my closet. I rubbed my bald head. Heaviness filled my chest. I cried, my pain seeping through tears as I considered my increasingly debilitated state. Like an opened floodgate, I trembled and wept uncontrollably. Streams of tears dribbled down to my mouth. Tasting salt, I reached for Kleenex after Kleenex, unable to mop up the physical and emotional spill. *What am I supposed to do with my life?*

Fifteen minutes later, I was exhausted, my cathartic release over. I hadn't cried that hard since I was a baby. The cancer experience was bringing me to depths of my core and emotions I hadn't experienced before. It was making me see myself from new angles.

It was my third day after the latest round of chemo, 11:00 a.m. I sat in a maroon swivel chair at my old desk, resting my elbows on my knees, wondering when the feeling of nausea would dissipate. Leaning back, I flashed to when this chair sat in my old condo and my heart tinged with sadness. I remembered myself healthy. This piece of my past, living in my condo, felt like it had happened years ago. The reality was it was only months prior. My mind circled back to the listless feeling and I contemplated whether I should call Dr. Mahdavi's office. I was still having trouble keeping food and fluids down. I needed a hydration IV.

Finally, I grabbed the cordless phone, dialed the office number, and asked to speak with Nurse Rebecca.

"Hi Christine. What's up?" she said, sounding hurried.

"Well, again I've been unable to keep fluids down for the last two days. I think I need a hydration IV."

"Come on in."

I hung up. Instantly, a hurling motion rattled my stomach. I grabbed my abdomen and quickly bent over, my head facing the floor. My stomach convulsed, but nothing came out.

After dry heaving for a minute, I walked to the bathroom and spit saliva into the sink. Patients for whom I'd cared on the BMT unit came to mind, particularly those who'd instantly thrown up when I entered the room carrying a chemo bag.

A phenomenon I hadn't really understood was now crystal clear.[15] I thought back to a patient I'd had eight years earlier.

Fluorescent lights shone down on shiny white floors in the halls of the BMT unit. As I passed by rooms, I noticed the bright summer morning outside.

Wearing a white dress uniform and white nursing shoes, I walked into Allison's single-bed room carrying an IV antibiotic. IV tubing dangled near my waist, as if I were carrying a purse. Allison, a thirty-five-year-old mother, had a narrow face and mousy features that seemed to match her personality.

Her hair looked like a thin brown helmet. She'd received high-dose chemotherapy from me the day before. This was a day of rest with no chemo, just IV fluids before her bone marrow transplant the following day.

With glazed eyes, she sat in bed staring at the cards and photos pinned on the bulletin board across from her. She turned to look at me in the doorway and began dry heaving. The sound of her retching was loud and dramatic.

I ran toward her and grabbed a kidney-shaped gold emesis basin from the bedside table, placing it under her mouth. She grasped the pan with one shaking hand and held her stomach with the other.

"Oh, goodness," I said, helping hold the basin for her. I patted her back, feeling sad for her. "Well, the chemo is working."

A minute later, she stopped.

I handed her tissues. She dabbed her tear-filled eyes. "I wasn't even nauseous," she said, clearing her throat. "It just came out of nowhere."

"That's what we call anticipatory nausea and vomiting, also called white-coat syndrome," I said, with regret. "Sometimes when patients see doctors or nurses, they throw up or dry heave. We're a trigger of unpleasant memories and trauma."

She spat out saliva in a tissue. "Don't take it personally."

I smiled and chuckled. "Trust me, I don't."

Now my turn, I dried my mouth off with a towel. So much of my life was out of control. Resting my hands on the bathroom counter, I drew my face closer to the mirror. I smirked at the reflection, finding humor in my reaction. *So this is what it feels like to be on the other side?*

Chapter 13

Blessings in Battle

There were times I tried to pray, but felt I couldn't even do that. Thankfully, God sent an army to help me.

Coastal fog and clouds left a palpable thickness in the afternoon air. My mom and Karen met me at Skylar's house, and then we drove to a wig store. It was on a busy street I traveled almost daily. Surprisingly, I'd never noticed the store before; I'd never needed it.

We parked the car and walked into what looked like an old-fashioned beauty salon. Lace curtains hung in the windows, and mannequin heads with long eyelashes stared toward the street, different wig styles atop their Styrofoam heads.

I opened the shop's white door and heard a bell jingle. The shop smelled like an elderly person's home. Toward the back of the barn-sized room was a barber's chair with gold-toned fancy metal on the footrest and above the cushioned back. The room's pale orange walls wore deteriorating paint that looked ready to chip off any day. Even though it was tattered in spots, the place felt homey.

We passed tables adorned with white lace doilies topped with fashionable hair accessories. Brown mounted shelves were stacked with the Styrofoam heads wearing wigs.

"I feel like I'm in a grandma's house," I said, noticing the creak in the wooden floorboards.

"This place definitely has character," Karen said, touching a short-haired auburn wig that sat on an antique-mirrored dresser.

"I'm pretty sure I know what I want." I pointed to a light brown colored, long, straight-haired wig. "I think I'm gonna try that one. Might as well get the hair I've always wanted."

"Why don't you see what it's like to be a redhead?" Karen asked with a chuckle, pointing to a neck-length fiery red wig.

"I don't think so. I want long, sexy hair."

A tanned sixty-something man with a blond mullet emerged from the back. "You ladies like to try one on?" he asked in a feminine voice, his smile adding crow's feet wrinkles to his hazel eyes.

"I'm the girl in need," I said, touching my pink polka-dot bandana on my head. "Maybe all us girls should try some on just for fun?"

"Sure. You'd be surprised who wears wigs," he said, picking up a head topped with a black wig that would make its wearer look like Joan Jett. He shook it and the shiny hair moved. "We make them look so natural. No one will know you're wearing a wig."

"These are beautiful," Mom said. "Are they made from real hair?"

"Some are." He took a wigged mannequin's head off the shelf. We stroked its hair.

"It's so soft," Karen said. "How long can one of these things last?"

"Well, it depends how much you wear it, but the real-hair ones can last over a year."

"I want to try that one," I said, pointing to the wig I'd seen initially.

He picked it up and escorted us to the barber's chair. I rested my arms on the chair's stiff sides as my mom and sister hovered nearby. I removed my bandana and he measured my head.

"I feel like I'm playing dress-up," I said with a giggle, peering into the mirror at my bald head.

Brushing the wig, he stood behind me and placed it snuggly on my scalp.

"This is the one," I said, smiling at myself in the mirror. I moved my head from side to side then held the hand-held mirror as he swung the chair around so I could look at all sides. *Pretty*. I remembered what it was like to be myself.

"The new me," I said, excited.

"Beautiful," My mom and sister said.

He removed the wig and I tied the bandana back on my head. We exited the store and I heard the jingle of the bell. Somehow I needed to try and not allow the cancer experience to suck out the essence of my femininity.

My wig wouldn't be ready for a few days. I sat on the living room couch feeling tired while waiting for Colin to come for a visit. My stamina and energy now fluctuated greatly from one day to the next. Leaning my head on the back of the couch, I gazed out the living room window and watched puffy clouds hover through tall pine trees in the neighbor's yard. I tried to look as presentable as possible in my red t-shirt and denim skirt, with a blue and white bandana covering my head, even though I felt self-conscious about not having hair or eyebrows.

I walked to the tile counter, rummaged through my purse, and applied pink lip gloss, hoping to add some color to my pale, gaunt face. In the bathroom, I inspected myself in the mirror. My eyes looked dull; I felt ugly. Exhausted from that task, I sat back on the couch, turned on the television, and closed my eyes. It took too much energy to care about what I looked like. Of anyone that should understand, it should be Colin.

The doorbell rang. Skylar answered it and escorted Colin to the living room.

"Hi Christine," Colin said, his tone sweet.

I opened my eyes and saw his strong, handsome face. He looked happy. He'd regained his muscular football-player physique. I grinned, getting a kick out of seeing him with messy, dark curly hair.

I stood and hugged him. His large frame held me tight. "I'm so glad you came."

"I'll go upstairs and leave you two to catch up," Skylar said.

As Skylar headed upstairs, Colin and I sat on the couch.

"I brought you something." Colin handed me a red Popsicle he'd taken out of the box. "I remember eating lots of these when I couldn't eat much else. The hells of chemotherapy." He rolled his eyes.

"Thanks." I grabbed the Popsicle and started licking it. "All I can think of to compare it to is when a train comes to a screeching halt. That sound of the ear-piercing friction and grinding of metal on metal." I gave him a disgusted look. "It feels like torture."

"There's no doubt, it is."

"Another thing that's unbelievable is how tired I am," I said, nestling my neck deeper into the couch and propping my feet on the coffee table. Colin did the same.

"Even talking is exhausting," Colin said, licking his Popsicle. "We don't even need to talk. Let's just kick back and veg on TV."

"I knew you'd get it."

Colin and I sat on the couch, watching re-runs of *The Brady Bunch* and eating our Popsicles. It helped to share my feelings with someone who'd been there. It comforted me. He didn't care what I looked like or what we did.

An hour later, he moved his focus from the television screen to me and said, "If only life was that easy."

I chuckled and gave him a smile. It meant everything knowing he was by my side.

Days later, I rested in bed with my eyes closed, listening to the crickets chirp on a warm night. Skylar was downstairs. I lay with a comforter and blanket piled on top of me, my body feeling as cold as a grocery-store cooler. Even though I hadn't received chemo in a week-and-a-half, I knew it was still ravaging me. What was this inner chill about? I'd taken my temperature and didn't have a fever.[16]

The flicker of light images changed on the TV screen in our dark bedroom. Chemo and all the weird things it does. I'd felt depressed and tired and had gone to bed at 8:00 p.m.

An hour later, the doorbell rang. When I opened my eyes, the bedroom door was ajar and the hallway light on. I heard Skylar clear his throat, then answer the door. I turned to lie on my side and lifted the sheet over my shoulders.

I heard the thud of his footsteps as he ascended the stairs. He stood in the doorway. "Honey, wake up," he said, enthusiasm in his voice.

"What's going on?"

"Come down and see something."

I took the carpeted steps down to the living room, holding the wooden rail. A six-foot tall artificial ficus tree sat at the base of the stairs, with what looked like a hundred yellow ribbons tied to the branches. Decorated as if it were a Christmas tree, each ribbon carried handwritten messages from the ER staff.

My eyes lit up and warmth filled my heart. "Wow!" I held one of the soft ribbons, reading the note. "I feel so special."

How fabulous of the ER staff! The news of my illness had spread like wildfire, also stretching to the PACU staff.

The generosity and caring was pouring in, as if I were a parched desert being hit by a monsoon. I'd received calls and cards from staff and friends saying they wanted to help, and that they were praying for my recovery. I couldn't speak with everyone who called, but I appreciated how they embraced me with love and kindness.

It was a sweltering September afternoon. Sitting in my car outside the building where I got lab work done every two weeks, I received a call on my cell phone. I looked at the number and left the car running so the cool air from the air-conditioner could blow against my face. Not recognizing the number, I answered.

"Christine...it's Dominique." Her voice was upbeat.

I was surprised but glad to hear from my boss.

"Just want you to know we miss you at work," she said, her voice sincere. "I have a surprise for you."

"That sounds fun."

"I know you're getting disability and that it's never the full amount of a paycheck," she said, delivering the information with her business-type voice. "So the ER staff and some others wanted to pitch in and help you."

Curious, I listened.

"We had a sign-up sheet for donating PTO (Paid Time Off) hours and people have been very generous." I pictured her sitting in her office wearing her signature pink pearl earrings and necklace, her face plastered with a smile. "I can't tell you who they are, but I can tell you they donated over two-hundred hours for you. I'll just say this: even the housekeeping and PACU staff wanted to participate."

"Wow!" I exclaimed. "Everyone has already been so giving. I deeply appreciate that."

When I hung up the phone, gratitude swelled my heart. I took in nature's beauty through my windshield, a light breeze tickled stands of green grass and tall eucalyptus tree branches delicately swayed. I thought of the other acts of kindness given to me. One such act came when paramedic/firefighters with whom I worked in the ER sent me flowers at home. The ER doctors contributed money and sent me a check to help with my expenses. One of the nurses told me her grandmother, who lived back east, was praying for me. Nurse Vanessa, the buxom, loud brunette with twenty years of experience in the ER, set her watch to beep the exact time I was receiving chemo so she could say a prayer of healing.

I shut off the car and walked into the lab, feeling grateful for the miraculous goodness in people. The kindness and caring from family, friends, and co-workers really uplifted me. Even though I was enduring one of the worst times in my life, I was also experiencing the most love I'd ever felt.

Chapter 14

MIND GAMES

It takes a lot of courage to step into the doctor's office to get chemo, especially when you know it's going to kick your butt.

The house creaked more than normal in the howling Santa Ana winds. It was the end of September and I was home alone. I stood in the kitchen, preparing for the next day. I felt unsettled yet industrious. I opened kitchen cabinets, pulling out supplies, my needed armor, to prepare for the fight my fourth chemo treatment would bring.

From one of the upper wooden cabinets, I grabbed five orange pill bottles. I lined them up on the tiled bar like toy soldiers, knowing each had its place in my defense against the side effects of chemo. I rubbed my thumb on the ridged white top of the Marinol bottle. Dr. Mahdavi had ordered it when I told him Zofran, Compazine, and Ativan weren't working very well to control my nausea. [17]

I opened the Marinol bottle and took out a hard amber-colored pill, massaging it between my fingers. I smiled surprised that a derivative of cannabis was in my arsenal of meds, but glad it worked against the nausea monster. I knew I'd be taking it after my chemo.

Another item in my arsenal sat on the bar: a six-inch tall porcelain angel with white wings, a white face, and a lilac-colored dress. One of the ER nurses gave it to me, saying she was the traveling angel of healing who was blessed by many people. My instructions: when I was better and didn't need her anymore, I was to pass her on to another person in need.

I put the Marinol pill back in the bottle and sat on the wooden barstool. Staring at the porcelain angel, I slid my fingers over her smooth golden halo. I said a prayer, but for some reason, didn't feel any connection. *Even more reason to be thankful for all the people praying for me.* I believed all their prayers had to be answered. My biggest Godsend and angel was Skylar.

I walked back into the kitchen, opened a lower cabinet, and took out two plastic bags. They rustled as I stuffed them into my purse. I would put one in the car, in case of an urgent vomiting episode.

My fingertips pulled at the shiny, metallic knob of another cabinet. As I grabbed a medium-sized Tupperware bowl and brought it into the living room, mid-morning rays of light shone through a small window. I placed it on the coffee table and thought how strange it was that I'd become accustomed to this way of life. My new job was to prepare myself for what lay ahead. No matter how much I prepared, I knew the hardest thing would be to protect my mental state.

From a wicker chair, I stared out the sliding glass door, watching strong winds bend bushes in every direction. Swirls of leaves blew across the patio. Some gusts frightened me with their power and noise. Like the chemo, I knew I would be bent by something strong. I anxiously drummed my finger on the arm of the chair. I looked down at my body, noticing a too-thin stomach and unhealthily bony arms. I'd lost fifteen pounds in two-and-a-half months. Prednisone makes many people gain weight. I experienced the opposite effect.

My mind spiraled out of control, preoccupied with what was to come. Tapping my legs, I felt uneasy, my heart beat faster, and I tasted sour saliva. *I never act like this. This is such a fucked-up situation.* Knowing I was starting to work myself up into a bad place, I got up and grabbed the Lance Armstrong book my sister had sent me. It was hard for me to understand my own mental state, but maybe the words of the world-class athlete who beat metastasized testicular cancer could shed some light on my emotional turmoil. I sat back down and opened it.

I read the first three pages of *It's Not About the Bike: My Journey Back to Life.* Tears streamed down my face as I read something that really struck a chord with me. It had to do with how cancer hits you from nowhere and slams you into a different life.[18]

I felt a sense of relief. The words connected to my soul and soothed me. It was monumental to me that someone knew how I felt and had made it through. I wiped tears with the back of my hand, and closed the book.

That night, I awoke in a panic, startled by a nightmare, gripping the cotton sheet with both hands. My heart raced.

Skylar was sleeping next to me. I sat up in bed and looked at the red numbers on the clock: 2:40 a.m.

The haze of the dream lifted into clarity: a robust, bald man with a voice full of hatred was robbing me. "Give it up," he yelled. "You're not going to win!"

A tug of war ensued. He wanted to steal my pink purse. I tried to hang on.

I pushed him forcefully with both hands. He stumbled, then whipped out a handgun from his heart. I crouched to the ground in defeat, fearful and helpless. I wrapped my arms around my head ...

Awake and in distress, I placed my cold hands on my face and shook my head, hoping to dismiss the horrible dream. Lying back on the pillow, I stared at the ceiling fan and listened to its rhythmic whirl. Skylar's sleeping breaths comforted me somewhat. I inhaled deeply and calmed down, my heartbeat returning to normal. Even in my dreams, cancer was pursuing me.[19]

I focused on the objects in the room, hoping to get past the dream and other things that plagued my mind. My eyes adjusted to the dark cracks in the closed wooden shades, allowing me to see hints of the moonlight. I scanned the nightstand, the dresser, two lamps, and a TV. All offered the small comfort of what was real and normal. Feeling the night chill, I pulled the comforter up to my chin and closed my eyes, hoping for a more peaceful sleep.

As any cancer patient can attest, processing your experience is often a case of one step forward, two steps back.

The next day, I leaned back in the seat of the SUV and put my elbow on the passenger door, resting my head on my knuckles. Skylar was driving up Pacific Coast Highway; we were enjoying a sunny morning. We passed grassy knolls, ritzy hotels, and people walking their dogs. The scenery offered a sense of calm I hoped would last all the way to the cancer center.

The four-lane road was busy. The radio played a mellow Jack Johnson tune as we passed familiar shops, gas stations, and street signs. I gazed out the passenger window and fixed my eyes on a man in a metallic blue Honda. He looked to be in his thirties, with a purple shirt and tie, and a stylish cut to his black hair. He held the steering wheel tightly, appearing hurried, determined. Along with the other drivers, he seemed to be speeding to work.

I was traveling for more chemo torture. Images of who I used to be clamored in my head: nurse, working person, independent, healthy. The relaxation I had experienced earlier now turned into anxiety. Visions of what the aftermath of my fourth treatment would be filled my mind. I swallowed often and tasted thick, sour saliva. Tears blurred my vision. Soon, I'd feel like I was at death's door.

The closer we got to the cancer center, the more distressed I became. I rolled up the sleeves of my pink cotton shirt and pushed the power window button down. I grasped the door handle as the wind blew strands of my wig.

"Are you okay?" Skylar asked.

I didn't answer.

"Just relax and take some deep breaths," Skylar said calmly. He patted my shoulder.

I tried to stop crying, but couldn't. The closer we got, the more I shuddered with fear. I had to keep this up for another four treatments? How could I keep this up?

"Try to calm down. It's gonna be okay."

Normally, Skylar's words comforted me. Not this time. The more I thought of what I was approaching, the more upset I became. I couldn't pull myself together. Instead, I fell apart, my emotions uncontrollable. My stomach tightened and convulsed. I started retching. I held my hands to my mouth. No vomit came out. Instead, saliva covered my palms.

Skylar pulled over. "Honey, you've gotta calm down and get a hold of yourself," he said with love.

I nodded and tried to breathe deeply as I heaved through sobs. As I dried my tears with the back of my hand, I focused on rubbing my thumbs together. *Okay, I can do this. Get a grip.*

Skylar put the car in gear and we continued our drive.

For a few minutes, I was able to look out the window at people walking near restaurants overlooking the bay. Then I started retching again. With an uncontrollable hurl of my stomach, I made a disgusting sound. I thought something would come up. I grabbed a plastic bag out of my purse, its rustling a familiar comfort, and rested it on my lap. The heaving continued, but nothing came up.

There was no logical reason for me to dry heave. My mind and body were taking over and doing crazy things. I hadn't undergone chemo in three weeks, but now that I was approaching my treatment, I was out of control.

We pulled into the cancer center parking lot. Skylar came to my side and opened the door. He nestled himself onto my seat, cradling my face in his hands. I broke his grip with my hands, buried my face in my palms, and wept.

A few minutes later, he grabbed a sweater from the backseat, and I dried off my face. "Honey, you've gotta do this. There's no choice," he said, his hazel eyes filled with sympathy.

I nodded. "I know." Sadness filled my voice.

He led me out of the car. With one arm around my shoulder and his other gripping my hand, Skylar steered me down the spacious hallway toward Dr. Mahdavi's office. I stared at the burnt orange carpet and walked cautiously. My emotional upheaval had left me deeply fearful.

Skylar opened the office door. While sobbing and attempting to take deep breaths, I knew this was not my usual way of entering. Normally, I'd write my name on the clipboard at the secretary's desk and sit in the waiting room for a few minutes. This time, I was escorted back to the chemo room immediately.

"Come with me," Nurse Rebecca said. Her voice sounded sad. I could tell she felt bad for me.

Looking down, I followed her white nurse's shoes and mauve scrub pants. Skylar helped seat me in a recliner, and eased into a chair next to me. I made sounds as if I were going to puke. Nurse Rebecca threw a gold emesis basin into my lap and a box of Kleenex into Skylar's hand. Tight fisted, I held onto both sides of the basin and dry heaved. A cacophony of sobs and dry heaving sounds followed. Skylar rubbed my back.

A minute later, Nurse Rebecca handed Skylar a cup of water, and my crying slowed. "Christine, take this when you're ready," she said, handing me a Valium.

Five minutes later, I stopped dry heaving and gulped the tablet down. I dried my puffy eyes and flushed face on tissues. I looked as if I'd been in a fifteen-round prize fight. How did I become such a basket case?

Skylar squeezed my hand. "Everything's gonna be okay."

There were three other patients in the room. One woman looked to be in her seventies. She wore a stylish short gray wig and dressy clothes. Her navy polyester pants and light blue silk top gave me the impression she should be heading into a corporate office.

"This is hard, but you can get through this," Ms. Stylish Seventy said in a kind voice, offering me a friendly expression. "We're all behind you."

I listened, embarrassed.

The only male patient was in his late sixties. His head appeared much larger and out of proportion to his skinny frame. He had pale blue eyes and thin lips that drew up into a smile. "We all understand how you feel," he said. "It's tough, but just think, after today is over, it's one last time you have to go through this."

I nodded, felt calmer, and wiped the last bits of tears from my eyes and blew my nose.

The other woman was perhaps in her late fifties. She wore a brown bandana and was knitting a turquoise blanket. "It takes a lot of courage to keep coming back in here," she said, as if she were my personal cheerleader. "We're all here for you."

I looked at each of them with my teary blue eyes and gave them a closed-mouth smile. I was touched by their concern.

Nurse Rebecca accessed my port. “Feel better?”

“Yep,” I said with a sigh, squeezing Skylar’s hand. “I don’t know what came over me. I’ve never acted like that before.”

“There’s no doubt, this isn’t easy to go through,” she said, starting my chemo.

Feeling emotionally lighter, I fell asleep.

Two hours into the infusion, I woke up. Looking around the room, I noticed Skylar wasn’t sitting in the chair next to me. He’d escaped for a break. I was glad he did. None of the other patients remained except Ms. Stylish Seventy.

“Glad you’re feeling better,” she said, catching my glance in her direction.

“Me too,” I said with relief. “I’ve never been that freaked out in my life.”

“It’s amazing the different hurdles life brings,” she said, scratching her wig. “What’s the saying? What doesn’t kill you makes you stronger.”

“That’s for sure.” We laughed.

Still feeling drowsy, I closed my eyes to reflect on what had happened. How ironic was it that oncology patients were now comforting me, when for years I’d been helping them through their misery.

After my four-hour chemo infusion, I felt more like myself. I headed into the office hallway toward the exit. Nurse Rebecca walked up to me, a serious look on her heavily made-up face. "Don't go yet...Dr. Mahdavi wants to see you in his office," she blurted.

Ugh. Go figure! It was clear my feelings and anxieties had been exposed. Now I'd have to talk to the boss.

She escorted me into one of the patient rooms. It was lunchtime and the office was closed. Since I'd been in the chemo room for a hydration IV during lunch, I knew some of the staff worked during this time. I hoped Dr. Mahdavi was in a hurry to have lunch himself and wouldn't take too long to talk to me. I wanted to get out the door as quickly as possible and forget about my behavior.

"Dr. Mahdavi will be right in," she said, and closed the exam room door quietly.

I took a deep breath, preparing for an anticipated lecture from Dr. Mahdavi. I was embarrassed about my emotional eruption in the chemo room. I pulled the neck of my cream-colored sweater closer, annoyed at why doctors' offices and hospitals had to be so cold. With my legs crossed, I rubbed my palms over my jeans nervously. Uncrossing my legs, I sat up straight, my attempt to look as put together as possible.

I scanned the room. It was familiar, the same room Skylar and I had occupied when we heard about my treatment plan. It was a typical doctor's office containing an exam table, a jar of tongue depressors, a blood pressure cuff, and a scale. The framed world map still hung on the wall. Disheartened, I looked at the map, remembering how I used to love traipsing around the world. Now my journeys were confined to my oncologist's office.

Dr. Mahdavi walked in, wearing a lab coat and a black stethoscope in one pocket. He closed the door and sat on a turquoise-colored stool, pulling it close to where I sat.

"I heard you had a hard time today," he said, his thick dark eyebrows raised in a question.

"I don't know what happened. I couldn't get control of myself." A knot welled up in my throat. I glanced at my white sandals. "My mind was playing tricks on me." My voice raised an octave and I giggled. "I guess I'm a bad patient."

He smoothed out his moustache with his fingers. "The only thing bad is the cancer that's in your body," he said sympathetically.

"This is so hard." I began to cry. "I don't think I can do this."

He wheeled the squeaky stool to the counter and pulled out tissues. Scooting the stool back to where I was, he handed them to me. "I believe it's harder going through this since you're a nurse."

I paused and looked into his coffee-colored eyes. It took me a few seconds before I saw the truth of his words.

"You've helped many patients through their journeys with cancer, never imagining you'd have to deal with it yourself."

Relief filled me. His insight was spot on. "I know too much."

"When patients have never dealt with cancer before, in a way, it's easier because it's all new. They don't know the treatments or what they're getting into," he said, his father-figure persona evident. "You've been an oncology nurse and have stood by patients through their cancer struggles. I'm sure it plagues your mind, knowing what you have to go through and thinking about what you've seen patients go through."

"Yes, it does."

"Your advantage is that you know the terminology and what's involved with cancer treatment," he said. "The disadvantage is you already know about the pain and trauma that's involved."

"So I gotta just forget what I know and wrap my head around this in a different way?"

Neither of us talked. His words settled further in my mind. I glanced at the world map and smiled. I needed to look at this as more of an adventure. A different type of adventure. And with more humor.

Dr. Mahdavi wrote on a prescription pad. "I think it'll be helpful for you to also be on an anti-depressant medication."

I laughed. *Great. Another pill. I'm getting used to this. Sign me up.*

Chapter 15

SUBMISSION

Seeing yourself in a debilitated state is a very humbling experience.

Two and a half days later, I awoke from a nap groggy and ambled over to the bedroom window. I stared out at the blue sky and heart-shaped birch tree leaves quivering from the mild breeze. Since my chemo room incident and talk with Dr. Mahdavi, I hadn't reflected on our conversation. Instead, my focus was trained on getting through the effects of chemo.

I staggered to the bathroom and stood on the oval-shaped white rug in front of the sink. I removed my light blue sweat pants, underwear, and white t-shirt top, allowing them to fall to the floor. I stared at my reflection in the mirror and felt the warmth of the overhead bathroom light. Sadness swept over me.

I leaned my hands on the hard edge of the marble sink. Tilting closer to the mirror, I inspected my pale bald head and sunken features. Heavy dark circles swooped below my eyes. My eyes looked lifeless. I had no eyebrows. Twisting my head to the right, I lifted my chin and noticed how grotesquely thin my neck was. Amidst taut muscles, my jugular vein looked as large as a hose. When I swallowed, the bulge of my Adam's apple became more pronounced, reminding me of a snake devouring a mouse.

Stepping back, I stood tall. I barely recognized myself. Grief filled me. I'd lost twenty pounds since my diagnosis. At first I was glad for a little weight loss, but not anymore. My collarbone looked like a thin tree branch jutting out from my upper chest. I rubbed my fingers over the bony structure and felt halfway around the bone. Moving my gaze below my left collarbone, I saw my Port-a-Cath sticking out, reminding me of something an alien would possess. I squeezed my protruding hipbones. Skin clung to bone as if it were cellophane. I hadn't an ounce of fat. Looking down at my pubic area, I saw no hair and was disturbed that I looked like a little girl. Layer by layer, cancer was changing me in uncountable ways.

I bent toward the ground and wiggled my fingers, trying to reach my toes. They looked as thin as a skeleton's, the definition of each toe bone outlined with skin. Unable to reach my ankles, I was frustrated – more reinforcement of how out of shape I was. Months of inactivity had taken its toll. Mortified, I stood up and put my clothes on.

I dragged myself back to bed. *What does Skylar see when he looks at me? Does he see me as another child to take care of and not his fiancée?* There was no hiding that I looked like a cancer patient; every aspect of my body—my life—had been devoured.

Two hours later, I awoke as our white bedroom walls faded to faint amber. The sun cast its final rays of daylight.

Feeling the need to pee, I headed into the bathroom. After I finished, I stood up. My head felt fuzzy. Black and white dots blanketed my vision and my legs were wobbly. I fainted.

Minutes later, Skylar roused me. "Honey, are you okay?" He sounded far away.

I blinked rapidly as I came back to consciousness. My arms and face felt the coolness of the linoleum floor. I pushed up to a sitting position and crossed my legs Indian style.

"Just sit there a minute," Skylar said, crouching down to eye level, looking concerned. "I heard a thud, so I ran up from the kitchen and found you plastered to the ground."

"I guess I just got up too fast," I said, rubbing my eyes. "I haven't had enough fluids today."

"Do I need to call the doctor and take you in?" He rubbed my back. "This is usually the day you need to head in for a hydration IV."

"I can't go back in there." I feared the chemo room trauma, and was unable to muster my sense of adventure.

Skylar pulled me to standing. "Honey, you gotta do what you gotta do."

I pushed past him. "I'll go downstairs. I need to take my pills, and I should try to eat something."

I cautiously walked downstairs and sat on the living room couch.

Skylar made me a quesadilla. I stood at the bar opening prescription bottles, putting pills into my palm. I picked up a glass of Gatorade and winced. *Definitely something I won't want to drink ever again when all this is over.* Nausea lurked. I caught a whiff of the bitter prednisone pill, and vomit inched its way upward. I ran to the toilet.

Five minutes later, I found my way back to the couch.

"I feel so weak," I said, curling into a ball and covering with a blanket. "I'm gonna call Tonya and see if she can come over. She'd said to call her if I needed anything. She can give me a hydration IV."

"She's offered numerous times, so take her up on it," Skylar said with a concerned look. He handed me my cell phone and sat next to me on the couch. "Luckily you know plenty of nurses."

For an instant, I felt bad imposing on my friend, and thought of her cat roaming her two-bedroom apartment. Desperate to feel better, I dialed Tonya's cell phone and left a message.

"I need an ER nurse stat," I said into the phone, in an attempt to lighten my mood.

I couldn't wait to hear back from her.

Even though exhausted, back in the spare bedroom at nearly midnight, I tried to stay awake and listen for Tonya's car to arrive after she finished her ER shift. I didn't have enough energy to look around and appreciate my old desk and things from my days before Skylar. I closed my eyes, hoping to find respite from the current difficulty in my life. I'd decided to sleep in one of the other bedrooms so Skylar could get a good night's sleep—and the smell of alcohol on his breath didn't help my feeling of nausea. The window was open. I was wrapped in a light blue sheet. A pleasant coastal coolness reached inland, and my thoughts went back nine months ago to my life in the ER. Tonya and I were working side by side. It was a fall evening and paramedics were wheeling a scraggly homeless man in by gurney. The white-haired, elderly man, who looked like Santa Claus, smiled and sang "New York, New York," while waving his arms.

A nurse walked by. "I didn't know Sinatra was singing here tonight."

"Quiet down," said the young, clean-cut medic, transferring him to the gurney. "I don't want you to scare other patients."

"Show tunes don't hurt anyone," he said, and continued his ballad.

Walking up to him, I looked into his gray eyes. "So, you seem very happy. What's your name?"

"My name's Mr. Jingle," he said with a grin, showing his yellow teeth. "Who are you, my dear?"

"I'm Christine, one of your nurses here in the ER."

"I get more than one?" His wiry white eyebrows rose.

"You sure do. Tonya is also your nurse," I said, smelling his horrid alcohol breath. I hooked him up to the EKG monitor and applied a blood pressure cuff to his arm.

Tonya's long lean body sauntered toward us.

I introduced them. "Two for the price of one. Hot dog!" He chuckled loudly.

Tonya looked at me, and we both smiled. We needed a little lightness after the seriousness of the past hour. We'd taken care of a heart attack patient who, after we treated him, had been whisked to the cardiac catheterization lab and then the intensive care unit.

An ER doctor walked up to Mr. Jingle and performed his assessment, writing orders for a banana bag (an IV bag containing special B vitamins and nutrients for alcohol toxicity). I obtained our needed supplies of lab tubes, an IV start kit, and an IV bag and arrived back at his bedside.

While hovering over him, Tonya and I tag-teamed performing our tasks.

"Are either of you married?" he asked.

"No," we replied in unison, giggling.

"Then I want to marry both of you!"

Tonya and I looked at each other, amused, and shook our heads. *Great,* I thought. *This is the offer I get - a man who's old, homeless, and drunk.* We laughed it off and then told Mr. Jingle he needed to speak in a quieter tone because there were other patients who didn't feel as good as he did. He complied for the most part, but continued to entertain us.

After our shift was over, we walked out the paramedic entrance and saw a parked ambulance and a starry night. While discussing our patients, Tonya said, "At least we got a proposal from Santa out of the day."

We laughed. I was glad to work with her. Together, we could tackle anything.

I opened my eyes and looked at the black stand-up lamp and its dull light. It was fun thinking about some crazy ER stories, but now my friend had another mission. I was hopeful Tonya's care and a hydration IV would nurse me back to life.

At last I heard a car door shut outside. Skylar was downstairs waiting for her. I closed my eyes, comforted that I'd soon feel more normal. The front door slammed, followed by the thud of footsteps heading upstairs. Tonya stood in the doorway wearing dark blue scrubs, a stethoscope poking out of her large purse. Her dark, straight hair hung to the sides of her long face.

"Christine, I'm here," she whispered.

I smiled faintly. "I'm so glad."

She walked closer. Skylar came up behind her and hoisted a bag of IV supplies onto the desk next to the bed. I'd gone to a specialty IV supply store the week prior, just in case, a part of my plan-ahead nurse mentality.

She scanned the room. "I'm gonna need somewhere to hang the IV. Can you bring the coat rack upstairs?" she asked Skylar.

I scooted over on the bed, and made room for her to sit.

"I'm not so perky right now," I said, my eyes stinging with exhaustion, my mouth dry. "I've thrown up three times today and can't drink that much."

"Just relax," she said in a calm tone.

Skylar placed the coat rack next to the bed. "Tonya, feel free to spend the night," he said. "We have the other spare bedroom." He pointed to the room next door.

Tonya agreed. I heard the fall of Skylar's footsteps as he walked downstairs.

"I think it's a relief for both of us you're here," I said, feeling her warm hands on my arm as she searched for a vein. Her touch soothed me.

"I'm honored to help you." Donning gloves, she put a tourniquet on my arm. "What are nurse friends for?" She opened an alcohol wipe and rubbed the back of my hand; her hands were like those of a skillful artist.

"Is your cat going to be okay?"

She smiled. "My roommate is taking care of Tazy."

I smelled the alcohol swab and felt its coolness on my arm. It was reassuring yet odd to have Tonya as my nurse. Being physically vulnerable brought me to new depths of humility and deeper levels of what caring should look like from a nurse and feel like as a patient.

My eyes felt heavy. "Let yourself relax and go to sleep," she said in a soothing lullaby tone. She inserted the needle and attached it to the hanging IV.

I closed my eyes. I never realized how difficult it was to be a patient.

She dimmed the light. "I'll check back on you." She closed the door halfway, and I heard her walk downstairs. While drifting off to sleep, I listened to Tonya and Skylar talk, their voices distant. I was grateful for my personal nurses.

Chapter 16

Some Things to Finish

It was a late Saturday afternoon when I drove down the black paved road, my mom sitting in the passenger seat. The sun's brightness reflected on palm leaves blowing in the wind, and branches of eucalyptus trees swayed leisurely. In a hurry since I'd left home late, I was anxious to get to my realtor's office. A low-level blah feeling had left me sluggish all day. Five days after chemo, the nasty feeling of nausea still wavered in and out. I pushed the accelerator, ready to sign the paperwork to sell my condo.

"It's a relief to get this off my back," I said, with a deep inhale. "Surprisingly, I don't really miss my condo."

"You had such a cute place." My mom patted my arm. "It's unfortunate, but the best thing."

"Glad I could sell it before I had to pay the three thousand dollar special assessment fee, which I don't have." I squeezed the steering wheel. "The association said there'd probably be more." I brushed strands of hair from my wig that had blown near my lips. "I'm glad it sold quick."

"You don't need that extra stress," Mom said, picking at a chipped nail.

The driver's window was a quarter of the way down. Wind turbulence mixed with music coming from the radio.

The breeze sent long strands of my wig hair flying toward the headrest. I rubbed my hairline and peeked into the rearview mirror, making sure I didn't need to readjust my wig.

Thankfully, I hadn't hit any red lights as we continued toward my realtor's office. Even though I felt like crap inside, I at least looked nice wearing a cotton pink print dress and beige wedge sandals.

"It seems like I was just going to Kamran's office to sign papers to buy my condo. That was three and a half years ago." I was touched with a hint of melancholy. "Kamran had told the buyer about the upcoming special assessment fees and he was okay with it. What a relief."

"You're doing the right thing," Mom said, embracing her tan cloth purse in her lap. "It'll feel good to have this financial stress off your back."

Suddenly, an uneasiness jolted my stomach. Clutching the steering wheel, I maneuvered to the side of the road.

"What's wrong?" Mom asked.

I couldn't answer. Reaching behind my seat, I grabbed a plastic bag and thrust it open below my mouth. I vomited the contents of my stomach, partially filling the bag. My eyes were wet with tears. My mom handed me some tissues, and I dabbed my eyes and wiped my mouth. I took a swig of water, swished it around my mouth, and opened the car door, spitting it on the black pavement.

My stomach stilled. I looked at my mom with wide eyes. "That was a surprise, a small detour in our plans."

"Are you sure you're okay?" Concern filled her face. "Why don't you let me drive?" Her shoulders looked tense.

"No, I'm good," I said, desperate to gain control of myself. "Gotta get back on the road. We're running late."

I'd driven another half-mile when the sick feeling returned. "Gotta throw up." I pulled to the curb and snatched the plastic bag behind my seat. I vomited again. "Great. Now I'm gonna smell like puke."

Mom rustled through the contents of her purse. "Oh gosh, I don't even have any gum. I'm so sorry you're feeling bad." A look of uneasiness crossed her face.

"I'm okay." I took some deep breaths.

We got back on the road, then had to pull over again. Twenty minutes later, we arrived at the realtor's office. After stopping the car, I peered at myself in the rearview mirror, and saw greenish-colored skin and bags under my eyes. In the big picture, selling my condo was nothing.

The ground-level realtor's office had a ceramic-tiled roof and glass front panels separated with beige columns. Miniature palm trees stood at the door's entrance. Mom and I walked up the concrete steps into the building. Combing my wig with my fingers and rubbing my tongue on my teeth, I hoped my breath didn't smell like vomit.

Kamran met us at the door. He was Persian, with a square head, mild voice, and thick dark hair. I liked him and his fun sense of humor; I could tell he cared about me as a client. I'd told Kamran I was undergoing cancer treatment. He hadn't seen me with a wig.

"Christine, come in. You look so beautiful," he said, fussing over me as he took my arm and led me to a chair.

"I'm sorry we're late."

"Don't even think about it." He brought us cups of water. "Are you ready to have your hand cramp?" he asked with a laugh, presenting me with a stack of papers to sign.

"Yep."

I signed the papers and handed over my spare key. I glanced at Mom. "Moving on with life," I said, relieved.

We left the office. My life as an independent single girl was now a thing of the past.

Chapter 17

Two Steps Forward, One Step Back

Each day was different. Sometimes, I felt different hour by hour. On the days when I felt more like myself, I wanted to venture out and attempt to do all I could.

One week later, I walked into Target with my mom. I was grateful for the cool blast of air-conditioning, a relief from the hot October afternoon. Bright lights illuminated the warehouse-sized store. My energy level was up. That made me happy, and I wanted to shop.

My brown flip-flops clicked to the stride of my steps as I passed rows of items ready for purchase. I held a red Swiss cheese-looking hand-basket. My mom tried to match my stride, but she was slightly slower.

She smiled. "You have those beautiful long legs. Remember mine are a lot shorter. Where do you want to go?"

"I'm feeling peppy. More normal." I matched her pace and wrapped my arm around her shoulder. "I need cotton balls. Let's head toward the cosmetic section."

We strolled down the long main aisle, and then cut into a shorter row filled with assorted body washes and lotions. I slowed my pace, out of breath. "I need to stop for a second."

"Take your time; we're not in any hurry," my mom said, her blue eyes filled with concern. She faked a smile.

I placed the red basket on the floor and grasped onto a beige metal shelf, my breaths feeling as if they were a teeter-totter. "I'm so tired."

"Maybe we should leave," she said.

"No, just give me a minute." I moved my gaze to the pomegranate body wash. I sipped in another breath. "Okay, I'm ready to shop."

We turned down the make-up aisle, looking at glossy lipsticks and eye make-up packages that were similar to a paint palette. Strolling down two more aisles, we reached the deodorants and cotton balls. My legs began to shake and my body felt exhausted.

"I need to stop again."

I lowered my body, crouching as if I were a frog. While balanced on my toes, I positioned my hands on the clean shiny floor. I bent my head forward, staring at my black shorts.

My mom stood next to me and acted like my bodyguard. "Just take your time."

I felt the stares of people passing by, but didn't look up. Mom patted my shoulder. *I'm the opposite of the energetic, bubbly person I used to be,* I thought. *I feel like an old lady.*

After a few minutes, I regained some energy. "How sad is that? I can't even walk down an aisle at Target."

"It's okay," she said, sadness quivering in her voice. "You have to consider all you're going through."

I straightened my legs, and slowly lifted myself to a standing position. "Chemo sucks," I said with a half-smile, tugging at the bottom of my shorts. "At least I have something to blame it on."

We left Target. I rested my head on the backrest of the car seat and closed my eyes. I felt weary, like I hadn't slept in months. *Remember, this is temporary, even if it feels like it's been six years.* I could hear myself repeating those words to my oncology patients, not realizing then what "tired" really looked and felt like.

Now I did.

On a mid-October evening, I entered the cancer center ready to attend my first cancer support group meeting. I wore a light sweater, jeans, and a blue and green striped top. I wanted to meet other women going through treatment and see how they lived with the demon. Another motivation was that my sister had told me she'd read an article stating that patients who attended support groups had better survival rates. Who doesn't want that? Armed with curiosity about how other women were dealing with cancer, I entered the building.

I opened the door to one of the meeting rooms, and fluffed up the sides of my strawberry blonde shoulder-length wig. One month before, I'd gone to the American Cancer Society and received a free wig. While wanting a different cut and color from my long light-brown colored wig, I'd figured I might as well have fun and try out new looks. I wanted adventure, right?

The room was air-conditioner cold, with off-white walls and a large square table surrounded by mauve cushioned seats. A whiteboard hung on one of the walls. Five women in their thirties sat in chairs. I joined them, thinking how sad it was we all had to be there. At the head of the table sat a smiling social worker in a pink suit and horn-rimmed glasses.

She started the meeting by welcoming us and asking us to tell our stories. An attractive African-American woman began speaking. She had a confident voice, chiseled cheekbones, and magazine-cover red lips. Her black-bob wig suited her features.

"I really try to make myself look attractive, even though there are days when I feel exhausted and horrible," she said, resting her hands on the table. "It's important for me to still look good for my husband."

The social worker asked, "What do you do to make yourself feel more attractive?"

"Well, I put on make-up and draw my eyebrows in with a pencil." A funny look came over her face as she mimicked her strokes. "It was helpful to go to the class the cancer center offers. It's called 'Look Good, Feel Better.' They give you tons of free make-up that companies donate. They have a facilitator who shows you tips on how to apply make-up. It was fun."

A few women in the group nodded their heads.

Another woman spoke up. Giselle was a larger gal with almond-shaped eyes and translucent skin. She wore a chestnut-colored wig with a turquoise barrette clamped on one side. The hair accessory looked as if it could be a child's.

"What's so hard is having the energy to go to work," she said, sharing glances with other group members. "I'm a single girl, so it's tough. I only have myself to rely on."

My heart ached for her. I was amazed she could go through cancer treatment without the support of a significant other. How thankful I was for Skylar!

"During the week, I come home and collapse on the couch, but on the weekends, I try to go out with friends. I even had a date," Giselle said with a wide smile. "Oh by the way, don't sit under an outdoor heat lamp when you're wearing a wig. It'll start to melt."

"Really?" a woman in the group asked.

"On the date my head felt really hot. I touched my hair and noticed a weird texture. I thought, *Oh my God, my hair's gonna sizzle right off.* What a date story," she said with an infectious laugh. "I told him I was cold and wanted to move indoors. Thankfully my hair didn't catch on fire, but I think it was close."

The group laughed.

Another woman hunched in her chair. She wore a purple oversized shirt and violet-colored bandana on her head. "I have two more months of chemo," she said, crossing her arms on her flat chest. "It feels like it's been forever, but I know I can get through it." With no eyebrows or eyelashes, she looked sullen. Her frail body and whispery voice reminded me of some patients I'd cared for in the oncology unit.

"It's funny how some friends called me when they heard about me having cancer." A forlorn look took over her face. "Then after the initial shock they stopped calling."

Many women in the room nodded.

"One person who I thought was a good friend didn't contact me at all."

I felt sad for her and knew the feeling. The same had happened to me. A friend of mine had heard about my diagnosis through a mutual friend. She never called or even sent a card. It hurt me, but I rationalized that some people just don't know how to react. Maybe it reminds them of their own mortality.

"It's helped coming here and listening to all of you," she said, a brighter look in her eyes. "It's good to know what I'm feeling is normal."

All the women were breast cancer patients. The hospital had another support group for all other types of cancer, but I was told the patients were sixty or older. I needed women my own age. The more I sat and listened, the more I felt a sense of camaraderie with these women. We were all young and struggling to make sense of our changed lives.

While leaving the group, I felt a sense of renewed hope, knowing others felt the same way I did. I stepped out into the starry night. Specks of light illuminated the darkness.

Days later, I sat on the couch with my hands clasped together and resting on my lap. Skylar was upstairs sleeping. I wore yellow pajama bottoms and a beige tank top as sunlight filtered into the living room. Birds chirped, announcing their happiness about the blue-sky Sunday, which was awakening with vibrancy and life. Hummingbirds whizzed in and out of a trimmed hedge in the backyard.

I wanted that same bright outlook. My plan the night before was to go to church, focus on God, and gain some sense of peace. Instead, fear and anxiety got the best of me.

When I wakened this morning, I'd felt a twinge in my left groin. I'd had some aches before, but this was more pulsating. Was the cancer worse? Did I have a new growth? Was the chemo not working? I looked around the room, scared.

On the bar, I saw my bottle of anti-depressant medication. My mind swirled into a dark place. My stomach clenched with fear. I touched my left groin again, wondering if I could feel lumps. Thankfully, there were none.

Ever since I'd started chemo, every twinge, headache, or soreness had made me question my body. I couldn't trust it. Sometimes, when I was past the throwing-up stage, just thinking about eating or drinking would make me anxious enough to dry heave. I'd never been a worrier. I used to be a live-in-the-moment, carefree person, but now it seemed I could never relax. It always felt like something was lurking over my shoulder. Cancer didn't just mess with my body, but also my mind.

I really wanted to go to church. I decided to go upstairs, shower, and get dressed. Skylar, who was half asleep, said he didn't want to go. I hoped being at church would comfort me. I figured God didn't ask me to go to church feeling good. He just wanted me there.

An hour later, I held a hymnal and listened to cheery piano and organ music play while the congregation sang. While singing every other line, I listened to off-key voices. I hadn't been going to the Presbyterian Church that long and only knew a few people. I felt self-conscious and alone.

After the hymn, the congregation sat. Nestling into the cushioned back pew, I looked around at the interior, an oval room with white walls and dark wooden beams in the ceiling. The church could seat three hundred people. The pulpit was elevated on three levels of carpeted stairs. Above the altar was a beautiful, very large stained-glass window. Many people surrounded me, but it didn't change my sorrow. I felt just as alone.

The pastor was forty-something, a clean-shaven man with boyish Midwest facial features. He wore a conservative brown suit and tie, and had a habit of touching his tie when he began his sermon.

"We can't always explain why bad things happen to us. Life can deliver some hard and unexpected blows."

I erupted into tears. I lifted my purse on my lap, and rummaged for tissues, dabbing my face. I inhaled deeply and lifted my head, seeing the cobalt blue and crimson cross in the stained-glass window. I looked back at the pastor as he said, "God can bring hope and peace in the most horrid circumstances." He scanned the congregation. "You might be saying, 'But you don't know how bad my situation is!' You're right, I don't." He seemed to stare in my direction. "But God knows and has a plan for your life. He can work all things for good for those who love God and are called according to His purpose."

I cried silently, releasing a gamut of emotions – fear, worry, anxiety, and the sense of the person I used to be. While sopping up tears on a tissue, I felt lighter. The room seemed brighter. Peace bathed my mind and soul.

The sermon ended. The song "It Is Well with My Soul" began. *When peace, like a river, attendeth my way, When sorrows like sea billows roll; Whatever my lot Thou hast taught me to say, It is well, it is well, with my soul.*

Joy consumed me. Hope began to blossom again.

Chapter 18

Relief in Knowing

An individual's entire community is changed by a cancer diagnosis.

The sun's warmth soothed my bare arms as I walked the hospital grounds, admiring the blue sky. The sun seemed to be shining more brightly than normal. Every bird, plant, and flower delighted me. I felt no apprehension about the reason for my visit, to get a CAT scan to assess how the cancer was responding to chemo. I was learning to stop worrying, to keep my mind in the present and to leave preoccupying thoughts to the wayside. This experience was bringing me an advanced lesson in mental training. I wanted to continue my day taking in life's goodness.

I stopped by the ER to see my co-workers before my visit to the radiology department. I wondered what they'd think about my new look – my long-haired light brown wig and twenty-pound weight loss. Dressed in camel-colored wedge heels, light blue Capri pants, and a V-neck sleeveless striped top, I felt confident as I grabbed the ER door and entered.

Patients of all ages were scattered around the rectangular lobby. A news show blared from the television, and a security guard stood at his podium near the back of the room. I spotted the triage nurse, Patrice. A feeling of melancholy came over me, remembering how I sat in the triage seat just four months earlier. I allowed myself to accept the feeling for a moment and then pushed it aside. I gave her a semi-circular wave.

Patrice's face lit up, and she motioned me over. She was a kind, heavy-set gal with the gift of making everyone feel special. She interrupted taking vital signs on a patient, stood up, and gave me a hug.

"It's so great to see you!" she exclaimed, looking me up and down. "You look so pretty."

"Thanks." I smiled and touched some strands of my wig. "Got a different look now."

"What are you doing here?" She sat and focused on starting the blood pressure machine.

"I want to say hi to everyone really quick. I have a CT scan next door in twenty minutes."

She buzzed me to the back.

I walked down a long pod with rows of patient-filled gurneys. Monitors beeped, and I heard recognizable voices of doctors and nurses behind curtain-drawn patient areas. The ER energy was invigorating. It still felt odd not working. I missed it. I continued my pace, knowing there was no way I could work a twelve-hour, stress-filled ER shift. I took in a deep sigh, remembering where I was in life for the time being.

I reached a wider area past the long hall and saw the central board with multi-colored patient names and information. To my right was an enclosed glass area where a few doctors and a secretary sat. Immediately, I was swarmed with a dozen nurses, doctors, and ER staff coming up to me for hugs.

"Christine, you look amazing," Dr. Nice said, greeting me with a soothing embrace.

"You guys are making me feel like a movie star," I said, elated with their affection.

"You look fabulous," Nurse Bridgett said. A beautiful redhead in bright pink lipstick. She was known for being able to start an IV on anybody. "We really miss you," she said, as another nurse pushed her away and gave me a bear hug.

"I miss you guys, too."

The word spread. More staff members gathered, doting over me with kind words and affirmations.

The crowd parted when Dominique, my boss, walked up. She'd come down from her upstairs office, after a secretary called her and told her I was visiting. Her navy pumps clicked on the white tile floor. She was dressed in a business suit and wore a cream-colored chiffon blouse, her signature pink pearls dangled from her ears and neck.

"Christine, I have to tell you what an inspiration you are to us," she said, her eyes welling up with tears. "You are a remarkable lady." She took two fingers and wiped the skin under her eyes, then gave me a solid hug.

"I'm so blessed to have all of you," I said, my heart swelling with gratitude. "It means so much, all your caring and prayers."

One of the nurses, Sissel, a striking blond, said, "We're definitely praying for you." She held her thin fingers together in the prayer position, her thumbs under the chain of her silver cross necklace.

"Thanks. Please keep praying. I'm going to get a CT after this," I said with hesitancy.

Nurse Bridgett left the group, then stepped back two minutes later. "Let me start your saline lock so you won't have to have the CT staff do it."[20]

"You're the expert."

She walked me to a back corner of the ER by the utility cart. I sat in a chair, and Bridgett started my saline lock. "It does my heart and head good to see everyone," I said.

"That reminds me, some of us girls are planning to take you to a pottery-painting outing whenever you feel up to it." She winked.

"Sounds like fun."

As I hugged Bridgett, I felt someone standing behind me. Releasing our embrace, I saw Tanner, the ER tech I had worked with regularly, standing with his arms crossed. His fingers tapped his upper arm, mimicking playing a keyboard.

"Like your new look," he said, uncrossing his arms.

"I like your new look, too." I smiled and reached up to rub stubble on his bald head. "When'd ya do that?"

"Tonya keeps us updated on you. She told me when you got your head shaved, so I thought I'd join the bald team." He gave me a charming look.

"Wow, you did that for me?"

"I figured I gave you so much crap at work, maybe I should start being nicer."

I laughed. "Awww."

"No seriously," he said. "I've been thinking. You should write a book." He gave me a tender look. "With all you've endured, I'm sure you have a lot to tell us."

"I'll think about it. Thanks." I pulled him in for a hug. "God knows I have a lot to write about."

I closed the door from the ER that led to a hallway carpeted in blue, and headed toward the radiology department. As I neared the entrance, I felt nervous, but then reminded myself of photos Tonya had given me from her recent trip to Tahiti. I thought of white-sand beaches and aqua-colored water, and knew I needed to put my mind in my happy place during the exam. I said a prayer, hoping my whole day would turn out perfectly.

Two days after my CT scan, orange light filtered into the bedroom through the slats in the blinds. Birds sang loudly. I sat up and stared at the fax machine across the room, wondering when the ER would send the report. A low-level fear haunted me. It had been easier to rest my mind in sleep than to be on pins and needles with anxiety about my CT results. I flipped on my stomach and put the pillow over my head, hoping sleep would continue to be my respite. So much for trying to be positive. I desperately wanted to hear the fax machine beep with the report, but instead heard a lawn mower from outside. My apprehension grew.

I lay back down, put the pillow over my head, and tried to think of other things. I listened to dogs bark, and then my mind turned back to worry. My stomach felt queasy with fear. I stared at the ceiling.

I'd never known how tortuous it was to wait for results. Now I did. Fortunately, while visiting my ER cohorts, one of them volunteered to look for the report, per my request. As soon as the radiologist read it, they would fax the results. Under normal circumstances, it might take my oncologist a week to get back to me. I felt such gratitude for my colleagues' help at every turn.

Unable to relax, I paced the bedroom, walking from the mirrored closet to Skylar's desk, where the fax machine sat. I stared at the receiver, examining every number and the illuminated red light. I glanced at numerous bills with the words "past due" lying on the desk. *That's strange. How could Skylar have let that happen?* Preoccupied with my inner turmoil, I dismissed the invoices, turned toward the closet, and saw myself in the mirror, frantic and disheveled.

My heart pounded harder, and my mind felt as if it were going to explode. *Oh my God, oh my God, oh my God.* I crouched to the ground in the prayer position, leaning my elbows on the bed.

"Please God. Please. Please!"

I stood, hearing only silence. My mental chatter nipped at me. Inhaling a deep breath, I felt embarrassed at how freaked out I was getting. *Get a grip.* I headed into the shower.

Fifteen minutes later, I tiptoed to the fax machine with a towel covering me. Three pages lay on the carrier. I smiled, finding humor and irony over how, in previous times when

I wanted something and was intently focused on it, it didn't happen. When I forgot about the thing I was stressing over and let go, it happened.

I picked up the pages and read the words: "A remarkable and significant improvement in adenopathy."[21]

The report discussed each tumor and location. All were significantly reduced by at least half.

I jumped up and down, elated. *Yes!* Just like that, I was one of the happiest women in the world.

Chapter 19

Bathed in Calm

I stood outside on cement slabs in the backyard, looking up at a dwindling sunset, a warm October evening. The sky had turned purple, adding to the beauty of the horizon. The orange clouds stretched out in a spider-web fashion. I appreciated the times when I could cherish nature's beauty. Satisfied with my evening visual, I reluctantly returned inside, knowing I needed to give myself injections of Neupogen and Epogen.[22]

As I walked into the kitchen, Skylar wore a preoccupied look as he braced his arms on the tiled counter. "What's going on?" I asked. "You look like something's on your mind."

"Ah, it's nothing." He pulled a vodka bottle from the top cupboard. "Got finances on my mind."

I looked away, unnerved he felt the need to drink so often. He had five or six drinks nearly every evening. Some mornings, he'd postpone business visits until the afternoon because he was hung-over. "Anything I can do?"

"Nah. Just work stuff."

I opened the refrigerator and took out packaged syringes.

"Time for your shot, huh?" Skylar put ice in a glass tumbler and poured vodka over it.

"Yeah."

I pushed my irritation aside. A flash of having cocktails with him at a restaurant came to mind. I'd thought he was just a social drinker, but in living with him, I saw things differently.

Who am I to say how someone should cope with cancer? "It's definitely been helpful being a nurse for this," I said with a smile, displaying the syringe in one hand. "I already know how to give shots." I started giggling. "Want one?"

"No, it's all yours, baby." He laughed and raised his glass to me.

I went to the living room and sat in a wicker chair, taking supplies out of a plastic bag. I removed an alcohol-wipe packet and laid it on the glass table. I opened the packed syringe, took off the cap, and tapped my middle finger on the glass, drawing the medicine upward and expelling an air bubble. A drop of liquid teetered on the top of the needle.

"You look professional over there," Skylar called from the kitchen, swirling his cocktail.

"I can't even count how many shots I've given to people. Hundreds." I lifted up my top and exposed my stomach, rubbing the alcohol wipe on a cushioned part. "It's kinda weird doing it on myself, but not a big deal."

Pinching some skin together, I injected the medication into my abdomen. After I gave myself both injections, I sat on the couch, and Skylar joined me. He wrapped his arm around my shoulder and we stared at the television.

I sat silently, uncomfortably. He reeked of alcohol. I looked through the sliding glass door at the white geraniums planted in the flowerbed, now fading in the encroaching darkness. Skylar had been so helpful and loving to me. *How can I complain?*

I nestled my head on his shoulder. *He's such a caring man. Everyone has some sort of problem in their life.*

I embraced him, feeling his warmth and comfort. I needed to be thankful for my moments of peace.

The next day, Skylar had gone to work late. I lay my head on a large couch cushion in the living room, holding my knees to my chest, trying to find a position of relief from the debilitating pain in my lower back.

The sun attempted to creep in through the closed brown shutters. The room was quiet, the television off. I had trouble keeping my eyes open and just wanted to drift off to sleep. I didn't have the energy to talk, nor did I want to.

My mom sat in a chair facing me, a look of worry on her face. "When's the last time you took a pain pill?"

"About ten minutes ago." I readjusted a heating pad on my back.

"Hopefully it'll kick in soon." She opened her purse and began sorting through its contents. "So Neupogen causes bone pain?"

I opened my eyes, irritated. "Yes."

"It's amazing how drugs have so many side effects," she blurted.

"Uh huh." I closed my eyelids, trying to shut out her noise and the throbbing deep pain. *Where was my escape-sleep?*

"I'll stay till Skylar gets home," she said.

Trying to suppress my annoyance, I said, "Mom, I really can't talk right now."

"Okay, honey."

I lay in stillness, reflecting on the hundreds of times I'd given my patients Neupogen. I couldn't recall any of them talking about how deep their pain was after receiving the drug. I remembered giving them pain medications, but never knew how depilated they might have felt. Had I walked into their rooms talking about whatever and not understanding they needed to rest?

Before drifting off to sleep, I raised my head to look at her. "Thanks for understanding."

She patted my crown with a soft touch. I felt the healing in quiet.

On a Sunday, days later, I sat with my mom on a beige church pew, rubbing my hands on the woven cushion. I craved the need for healing and soulful quiet—church. It had been sixteen years since I'd been to the Methodist Church I'd once attended.

We listened to the organist play "Peace Like a River." I looked up at the A-frame ceiling and its dark wood beams and saw blue sky filtering through the skylights. I moved my gaze to the front of the church, where square panels of colored stained glass depicted Jesus and his welcoming arms. I thought fondly of the time I had participated in the high school youth group, and of my boyfriend and other friends back then. I felt at home.

Coming out of my reflective state, I turned and looked toward the back of the church, noticing parents of friends from the youth group. They looked older than I remembered.

Some had aged well, others not. I was reminded of how much time had passed and the difficult things I had been through since I'd seen them last.

It left me feeling exposed. "Feels kinda weird to be back here after so many years," I whispered to my mom. She nodded, clasping the rolled-up church bulletin in one hand. Her bright blue eyes were soft, complemented by her pale pink lipstick. She looked relaxed. I liked seeing her that way.

The unfurling of past to present left me melancholy. I cleared my throat and held in the mountain of emotions that wanted to spill out. I wondered what people thought of seeing me after all these years.

Flipping open the church bulletin, I read a section in blue letters, the prayer requests. I scanned the names and saw mine. I swallowed deeply and closed the bulletin, surprised. The church had been helpful to my family in the past. When my dad was involved in that near-fatal car accident over twenty years earlier, he was hospitalized for three months. They sent food, cards, and many prayers. Now, their kindness had filtered to the present.

The pastor began speaking. A balding man, he wore square black-rimmed glasses, a gray suit and striped green and white tie. His voice was even, soothing. "I'd like to start off with praises," he said. "Anyone have any announcements of praise?"

Four people stood and said what they were thankful for.

"Now I'd like to ask if there is anyone who has a prayer request." He clasped his hands together, standing relaxed, as he scanned the congregation.

My eyes grew wide and I began playing with my fingernails. My heart beat at a rapid pace. I felt a squeeze from my mom's hand on my wrist.

The organist began to play.

"If you are hurting or need healing, can you please come to the altar?" he asked in a smooth tone, opening his arms.

She whispered, "Let's go up."

Nervous, I stood and walked to the altar, my heart beating faster with every step. The mood in the church was serious and focused. Others in need walked to the altar.

My mom followed me.

"James 5:14 tells us if any one of you is sick, you shall be anointed with oil and prayed over in the name of the Lord."

My legs wobbled as I reached the carpeted altar and knelt, grabbing the walnut handrail. Butterflies rumbled in my stomach.

The pastor stood in front of me and in a subdued voice asked what I needed prayer for.

"She has cancer," my mom sputtered, her voice cracked.

I clasped my hands in the prayer position, and watched the pastor. He took a small glass decanter of oil and dipped it on his thumb. I heard the rustle of people standing behind me and heard my mom sob, her shaky hand on my shoulder. The warmth of other hands rested on my shoulders and the back of my head. I closed my eyes and bowed my head, melting into their caring state. I felt the pressure of the pastor's thumb applying oil to my forehead and heard the people surrounding me say prayers.

"We pray for Christine's complete and total healing," the pastor said. "May these prayers, offered in faith, make her well."

Tears trickled down my cheeks as I felt an overwhelming peace. Thankfulness filled me for the care and help I received at every turn. I was aglow with God's spirit.

Days later, a faint breeze tickled my scalp as I climbed the stone inlaid steps toward the lab. I chuckled, surprised at how the breeze felt on my scalp. The sun peeked out of the clouds every so often, a reminder of the warm day transpiring. I stared self-consciously at every step my black flip flops took and wondered if people were looking at me. I'd made the decision to do some errands without wearing a wig, hat, or scarf. It was important to own who I'd become, yet I was curious how people might react. Though apprehensive, I didn't abandon my mission.

The building was square with offices in the perimeter and palm trees, grass, and stone benches in the center. Off-white stucco and fading brown trim revealed its age, its 1970s-style construction.

I reached the second floor walkway and lifted my head high, smiling at two passersby. They quickly looked away. Fear and embarrassment rushed inside me. I took a deep inhale and opened the door to the lab.

The lobby was the size of a closet and housed six vinyl chairs, one fake birch tree, a table with *People* magazines, and a television, which offered health information that sounded like an infomercial. It blared, but others in the room didn't seem to flinch at its annoyance.

Straightening my posture, I put on my most confident face and walked to the clipboard, hiding my insecurity. My heart beat in my throat and my pupils enlarged with the rush of adrenalin. I tamed my responses enough to appear calm.

I recognized the heavy brunette lab technician at the front desk. She wore a white lab coat that fit so tight on her arms it looked as if the seams would burst. She lifted her head and looked at me; her silver-rimmed glasses magnified her thick lashes. She paused and gave me an odd look, then started talking to me as we normally did.

"How ya doing today?"

"I'm feeling good," I said, watching her peer at her paperwork.

She'd drawn my labs countless times. She and another technician seemed to be the only full-time employees. When I'd sit in the lobby, waiting to go in, I felt sympathy for them, even though the forty-five minute wait was annoying. As is typical in the medical profession, the staff works hard and there's usually an understaffing issue.

I sat in the wood-framed turquoise chair, watching patients flip through magazines. Some slumped in their chairs. I occasionally glanced at the obnoxious television program.

An elderly Hispanic gentleman sat across from me. He had white hair and moustache and leaned on his clubbed cane. Looking up, he offered a pleasant smile. I returned his smile, happy he'd given me a boost of confidence.

I leaned my elbow on the armrest, and scanned the room. In the corner sat a tall, thin man with a beakish nose and kind face. A cast covered the lower part of his right leg, his plaster-dusted toes exposed. He gave me a likeable look.

"What happened to your leg?" I asked.

"Oh, I broke a few bones skiing," he said, with a deep sigh. "Then at a freakish fire pit accident, I got a burn on my upper arm. I guess the injury was so traumatic I needed a skin graft from my upper thigh." He looked down with disgust at his upper leg, now wrapped in a bandage. "Such a nuisance."

"I bet. I'm sure you're ready to be healed and have it all over with."

"To say the least."

"I know the feeling." We laughed.

The entrance door opened and another patient walked in, a middle-aged heavy-set businessman who wore khaki trousers and a blue shirt with pit stains. His blond hair was in a crew cut, and he had a sparse beard. He grimaced when he looked my way, and his eyes quickly darted away. I sensed his uncomfortable awkwardness over my exposing my illness, not covering it up. I was an oddity in a normal world used to seeing something else. I realized that observing a person who doesn't "look right" causes fear and discomfort. It rattles thoughts of order and how the world should be.

After waiting thirty minutes, the interior door opened. "Christine, you can come back," the other lab technician said. She held open the door for me to enter.

Kimberly was young with an angular face and scraggly blond-hair. On many of my previous visits, we'd talk about nursing and nursing school. She was taking prerequisites and waiting to get into a program.

"Hi," I said in a cheery voice, feeling like I was seeing an old friend.

I towered over her small frame as we walked to one of the lab rooms. Moving my head from side to side, I found it unusual not to have my wig rub the back of my neck. Unlike previous visits, there was a long lapse in our conversation. I sensed she was caught off guard and didn't know what to say.

I sat in a plastic orange chair and hoisted my arm on the college-sized half desk. Lab tubes of assorted colors filled white plastic phlebotomy trays. Alcohol wipes and tourniquets were stacked next to the tubes.

"Busy day again for you girls, huh?"

Her gaze slowly moved to my face.

"I'm trying a different look today," I said, relieved to break the ice. "It's an experiment."

"Going natural, huh?" she asked, with a shy hesitancy.

"Yeah, I thought why not?" I exuded a happy tone. "Have some fun with all this. Experience life as a bald woman."

"You're so daring."

"Why be fearful?" I closed my fist as she applied the tourniquet. "I've traveled lots and been on many adventures, so I figured I'm going to make this an adventure."

"I think that's great." She wiped alcohol on my antecubital area (bend of the elbow). "You're a brave woman. I don't think I could do that."

"Gotta live life and try new things." I felt the needle prick my arm. "I'm gonna go to Sav-On after this and see how it goes."

She filled lavender-, blue-, and red-top tubes with blood, then released the tourniquet while applying a cotton ball.

She grinned.

"I'll be interested to hear your final analysis."

As I stepped out of the lab, the sun burned through the edges of a cloud. I smiled, happy to have accomplished my mission. Even though some things in life can be off-putting and difficult to look at, it's worth it to push past the discomfort and offer a compassionate smile. *You never know who'll be watching and what they might learn.*

I entered the solid structure of the First Presbyterian Church, tousled by the strong winds blowing outside. Once in the foyer, I brushed the strands of my wig with my fingers and felt a few tangles. I straightened my wig and re-adjusted my coconut-colored cap-sleeved top, questioning whether my decision to attend the Bible study was a good idea. I was a Christian, but hadn't always lived the most Godly life.

I walked into the interior of the church to meet a group of ladies for a study on Ephesians. I was unsure if I was knowledgeable or spiritual enough to be part of the study, but knew my soul needed recharging. With encouragement from my new friend Lorraine, I decided to attend. Normally, I was excited about meeting new people, but this time I felt nervous. All of the downtime left me feeling lost. I decided it would be a good investment of my time to meet spiritual women and deepen my connection with God.

I was matched up with Lorraine in a church program called the Stephen Ministry. The program partnered someone going through a crisis in their life, with someone with spiritual wisdom who was a good listener. She'd taken special training to become a volunteer in the program.

Though seventy, Lorraine had the looks and body of a forty-year-old. Her blond hair was cut short, framing her petite face, which accented her green eyes and beautiful smile. She practiced yoga three days a week and was filled with high energy and a spunky attitude. Her words and actions were grounded in a deep faith that intrigued me. She was on my side, helping me with prayer and wisdom. The cancer experience and her amazing spirit made me want to deepen my faith.

I stood hand in hand, praying with other women in the Bible study, feeling light-headed. Sometimes, abnormal feelings in my body occurred for reasons I couldn't explain. Opening my eyes, I looked at the beige carpet and the steps toward the altar, trying to regain my stability. The leader of the group prayed for people in need, me included. Even though my mind wasn't completely focused, I hoped all our prayers would be heard and answered.

I gripped Lorraine's hand. I couldn't help but lean into her short frame, hoping I wouldn't drop to the floor. I felt her weight hold me up. She gave me a concerned glance. The praying ended and I eased onto my folding chair.

I whispered to her in her left ear, surprised she had a hearing aid. "I almost fainted."

"I could tell. We can step out if you'd like. Do you need some water?"

I pulled out a water bottle from my purse. "I'm okay."

The Bible study continued for another ten minutes. When it adjourned, Lorraine said, "Let's go to lunch."

While driving to the Mexican restaurant, I reviewed how much upheaval and change I'd experienced. Cancer made me question everything about myself and how I coped with life. *Had I been eating the wrong foods? What did I do to deserve this? Should my life take a new direction?*

I pulled up to the restaurant and met Lorraine. I knew I didn't have the answers, but hoped I would emerge from all this with more insight about my life.

We placed our orders, nibbled on salty chips, and drank bitter iced tea. "I have something for you," Lorraine said, pulling out a gray and purple afghan from a Nordstrom bag. "My ninety-year-old mother made it." She smiled brightly. "All day she prays and crochets," she laughed. "Proof that God has use for us even when we're old."

She handed me the afghan and I placed it in my lap, petting the soft material. "I'm so honored."

"Sometimes God uses tragedy to grow us," she said, looking intently into my eyes. "Like a needed operation, we don't want to get cut open or go through pain. It can be frustrating, the time and patience involved in healing, but that's what's needed."

I nodded, taking in her words. I thought I knew a lot as an oncology nurse, with my bedside view of cancer. Like a pendulum, though, life had swung me in a new direction of understanding. I hoped my new perspective would offer greater meaning to others in the future.

The food arrived. Lorraine reached over and squeezed my hand. With a sparkle in her eyes and a wide smile, she said, "If you stick close to God, I think some day you're going to be amazed at how He's going to orchestrate your future."

Chapter 20

More Change

The frustrating part is there are so many steps in this escalating experience.

Dressed in jeans, a tank top, and a light blue cardigan, I opened the heavy door to Dr. Mahdavi's office with a sense of determination. The week before, I'd received my fifth chemo, and was now at an office visit and Rituxan treatment, which followed one week later.

For a couple of weeks, I'd thought about my second opinion visit in July with Dr. Prism. She'd told me her hospital gives chemo and Rituxan on the same day. Tired of coming into Dr. Mahdavi's office so often, I wanted to alter my treatment plan. With strong intentions of convincing Dr. Mahdavi, I equipped myself with a clear mind and purposeful energy.

I entered the office, wrote my name on the clipboard, and sat in the waiting room with crossed legs, nervously shaking my top foot as if I were a tap dancer. One of the nurses escorted me to an exam room, where I parked myself on an uncomfortable orange vinyl chair. While rehearsing my talking points, I noticed two small hanging photographs of cherry blossoms on the eggshell-colored wall. I remembered years before, when I'd gone to Washington, D.C., and seen cherry blossoms on hundreds of trees. The Japanese associate them with mortality because of their extreme beauty and quick death. I quickly looked away and flushed negative thoughts out of my mind. With perfect posture and hands crossed in my lap, I put on a cheery face when I heard the doorknob turn.

Dr. Mahdavi entered the room and gave me a closed-mouth smile. He sat on a squeaky stool and flipped open my manila chart. I stared at his name, stitched in blue cursive letters on his lab coat.

"You're looking happy today," he said. He briefly studied the paperwork. "I like seeing that."

"Thanks," I said, in a shy tone, trying to gain confidence again.

"You've finished your fifth chemo and are going to get Rituxan today." He looked away from his paperwork and up at me. He conveyed calmness as always.

"Yep. I'm glad I was only sick one day after the fifth treatment," I said with a hearty smile. "What a relief."

"Good." His fatherly persona soothed me. "As we saw from your CT scan, the chemo is working nicely. Initially I told you you'd need six or eight treatments." He paused and smoothed out his salt and pepper moustache. "I'd like you to have eight."

I felt as if an electrical jolt had hit me. "Ugh," I replied, frustrated. "Are you sure?"

"I want to be as certain as I can that the cancer is completely gone and won't come back," he said, confirmation in his voice. "Eight treatments is what I want you to have." He gave me a stern look.

I sighed. "I'll do whatever you want." Deflated, I paused. "I need to ask you something."

He closed the chart and rested his arms on his legs. "What would you like to talk about?" He raised his thick eyebrows.

I inhaled deeply, gaining my courage. "I want you to use me as a guinea pig," I said, pleading in my voice. "You probably weren't happy that I had a second opinion." I spoke quickly, leaning toward him. "It's not that I didn't trust you. It just put my mind more at ease. I used to work there."

"I remember." He sighed and clasped his hands together in the power position. "Go on."

"Well, when I spoke with Dr. Prism, she said they give chemo and Rituxan on the same day." I looked to the ground and then peered into his serious face. "I'd like to have you try that on me."

He gazed down at the carpet and said nothing.

My heart beat fast, afraid I'd insulted him. As an uncomfortable silence began to spread, I said, "Please Dr. Mahdavi." I put my hands in the prayer position. "Please, I'd really just rather get it all done in one day every three weeks than have to come for Rituxan the week after chemo." I felt as if I were a lawyer pleading my case or a child begging a parent for candy. "I've had no problems with Rituxan. Please let me try it."

"Well..." His silence seemed to last an hour. "Okay, we'll try it on your sixth round."

Jumping up with excitement, I threw my hands around his neck and pulled him in for a hug. "Really, it's gonna work out." I released my grip. "Thank you so much."

He walked toward the door, shutting it carefully behind him. I was glad I acted on my conviction. Pumping my fists in victory, I hoped to continue on this trajectory of things getting better.

A week later, I stared out the window of gynecologist Dr. Kroll's waiting room, watching wispy clouds accent the afternoon sky. I had taken Dr. Mahdavi's advice to see my gynecologist because I was experiencing hot flashes. The large fifth-floor window looked out to palm trees, buildings, and a car-filled parking lot. I enjoyed the elevated view and felt removed from the realities of my life. Until I scanned the lobby.

Seven pregnant women scattered around the room, cradling their large bellies. Another woman and I were the only apparently non-pregnant ones. I picked up a *Travel and Leisure* magazine from the enormous coffee table and flipped through the pages. I felt alienated, wondering when my life would turn out like I wanted, which would include a husband and a child. I took in a deep breath and glanced down at the engagement ring on my finger. I remembered the conversation Skylar and I had in Spain. He'd said when the time was right, he'd have a child with me. I brushed off my baby cravings, and hoped to be called to an exam room soon.

A medical assistant escorted me back, and I changed into a pale blue paper gown. I sat on the cushioned teal exam table, making crackling sounds with every little movement. Attempting to soothe my fears about what was happening with my body, I played with the long strands of my wig. I eyed the folded metal stirrups on each side of my thighs and hoped I wouldn't need one of those exams today.

Dr. Kroll entered the room. She was a petite blonde with Scandinavian features. I'd taken care of some of her patients when I worked in the PACU. I loved her bedside manner and how sweet and caring she was to her patients, including me. Throughout the six years she'd been my doctor, she'd looked more like a college girl than a gynecologist. She always seemed to genuinely care about me, almost as if I were a friend.

"Hi! So glad to see you!" she exclaimed in her raspy jazz singer voice. She scooped me into an embrace. "You look beautiful."

"Thanks."

She sat on a metal-based stool, pulling it close, practically under my legs. "So, I have to say, I was absolutely shocked about your diagnosis. How are you dealing with all this?"

"Well, it's been quite an interesting adventure," I said, rolling my eyes. "But I guess it's making me a stronger person for whatever else that's gonna happen in my life."

"Look how amazing you are." Her crystal blue eyes twinkled. "You have such a positive outlook."

"All I can do is keep getting through it all." I flashed a half-smile. "At least now I know what women feel like when they complain about hot flashes." I laughed.

"No need to be burdened with that," she said in a sympathetic tone. "I got your lab results." She opened a manila-colored chart. "You're in full-blown menopause. No wonder you're feeling the way you are."[23]

My eyes widened. I gulped hard.

"So what do we do about it?"

"I'm writing you a prescription for a hormone, an estrogen replacement therapy called Activella. With all you have going on, you don't need to be burdened with hot flashes."

"Is it okay for me to be on a hormone?"

"Since you don't have breast cancer, it's safe for you to take it temporarily."

I looked down at my chipped pink toenails, feeling uneasy about my other looming question. "So do you think my period will come back? I...I'd like to have kids someday."

"When you finish chemo, and your body has a chance to regroup, I would expect you to reverse out of it." She cleared her throat; a clinical look took over her face. "But there's no guarantee."

I stared at a jar of cotton balls on the sink and took a deep breath. This whole process had been about changes and not knowing what the future held. I needed to let that piece of the puzzle go. "No sense in me worrying about it," I said, with resolve.

We hugged each other as I prepared to leave.

I stepped out of the building and walked to my car while looking up at the sky. The wispy clouds had disappeared. A breeze tickled my bare arms. Sitting in the driver's seat, I thought about my view from the window upstairs compared to that of the windshield of the Mercedes parked in front of me. I had no idea what was ahead of me on this journey. The only thing I could do was look at my circumstances with a perspective of humor and faith that someday things would be better.

Peering out the sliding glass door window, a week later, I watched the wind scatter sycamore leaves across the patio. Branches of large juniper bushes bent at the mercy of strong gusts, reminding me of my body's struggle through chemotherapy.

Skylar stood in the kitchen drinking coffee and turning the pages of the newspaper. I sat at the bar overlooking the kitchen, eating breakfast, delighted to be feeling well. "I'm so thrilled I didn't get sick after my sixth chemo treatment," I said, scratching my head, feeling the soft bandana. "Maybe I'm onto something with having the Rituxan the same day?"

"I'm sure Dr. Mahdavi will send you a check for helping him come up with that plan," Skylar said with a snicker.

I brushed off his comment finding it odd, and said, "I want to do something fun today. Let's take a walk on the beach." I forked scrambled eggs into my mouth.

Skylar's hazel eyes peeked over his reading glasses at me. He was attractive with his gray morning scruff. "I'd like to go look at houses."

That shocked me. "What?"

"I've been thinking it'd be nice to move to a different place." His hands were braced on the counter. He stood directly across from me. "You could invest the money you got from your condo."

My happiness immediately turned into discomfort. "I didn't have any idea you were thinking of moving," I said. "What's going on?"

He gazed down at the sink and sighed. He looked disgusted. "This place is my ex-wife's, and she wants to sell it."

I swallowed hard, feeling confused. Confrontation wasn't one of my strong suits, but I needed to say it. "I thought you owned this place and I was helping you out with the mortgage?" I had been giving him money for expenses since I'd moved in with Skylar. That was the least I could do, considering all he was doing for me.

"I fell on some rough times a while back. She helped me out."

"That was nice of her," I said, trying to wrap my head around the news. How odd that he was fifty-eight and still not financially secure, especially since he was an investment advisor. I remembered how he used to love spending money wining and dining me.

A sense of betrayal filled me. *Had he lied to me?*

"We could buy a house and use your money as a down payment," he said, folding the newspaper.

Suddenly, I felt hurt and pressured. "I don't want to make any major decisions or purchases. I have enough going on right now." I walked to the sink and rinsed off my plate. "I'm a little gun-shy just getting out of my condo and all that happened with that."

He threw down the paper and stormed off.

I sat on the living room sofa and stared absently at the swaying juniper bushes. Now shaken, I pondered how little Skylar had told me about his life. Nothing in my life felt secure.

I drove north on the 405 Freeway toward my sister's house in Montrose, about an hour away. With all the changes going on, I craved stability and was glad to be heading to family. The prospects of menopause and the issues with Skylar left me mentally fatigued. Spending time with my sister and nieces would lift my spirits.

I wore my strawberry-blond shoulder-length wig and sat on the living room couch at my sister's house, cuddling my four-and seven-year-old nieces. The house was a charming 1940s style with a door-slotted mailbox and white rectangle-tiled kitchen. After snapping a photo of my nieces and me, my sister walked across the creaky wooden floor and sat on an oversized striped chair. It was early evening and she'd changed into flannel pajamas, her chestnut-colored hair in pigtails.

"Let's get this party started," she exclaimed. She walked to the CD player, and turned on Michael Jackson's song "Beat It".

Wearing princess-print pajamas, my nieces scurried to the oval rug on the living room floor and began jumping up and down, their blond hair bouncing. "Come on Auntie, get up!" the seven-year-old said. They ran to me and pulled me up by my arms.

"I'm ready." I shook my hips to the beat.

The four of us shimmied and jiggled our bodies, laughing.

During the chorus we all sang, "Beat it." I pointed my index finger up, feeling as if I were telling the cancer that I was going to win. Happy and free of concern, I pulled off my wig and twirled it around in a circular motion as if I were a cowboy in a rodeo. Their poodle barked and circled. "Woo Hoo!" I exclaimed.

My nieces screamed with glee, and my sister bent over in a deep belly laugh.

"Auntie!" They yelled and ran over to hug me. The song ended, and they grabbed my wig, each putting it on their heads, showing their best model poses. They placed it on the poodle's head and said, "She likes it," as the dog scratched to get it off.

I watched, entertained by their giggling and amusement, now feeling carefree and happy, I was delighted by the love and silliness that only a child can bring.

Chapter 21

Mountain Top

Bright morning sunlight filtered into the chemo room and the December sky was an eye-piercing blue. I sat in my recliner, wearing a butterfly capped-sleeve top that matched my upbeat mood. Nurse Rebecca hung a sandwich-bag-sized IV of Zinecard on my IV pole after I'd gotten my chemo.[24]

"Have I been getting this every time?" I asked.

"Yes, Christine." She sounded irritated, implying I should know.

"I guess I've been so out of it during the other rounds, I didn't notice," I said apologetically. I thought about my previous times in the chemo room and reflected on my irritation when I'd had a difficult patient. Had I been one of those?

She took a patient's blood pressure and walked out.

I felt like chatting. I looked at the only other patient in the room, a woman in her seventies who wore attractive business clothing and a smoke-colored wig in a short bob. It was Ms. Stylish Seventy, the woman to whom I'd talked months earlier when I'd entered the room crying and anxious. Reclined in her chemo chair, her IV line was tucked under her collared shirt. She projected a confident attitude. Thankfully, this time I was in a jovial mood.

I smiled. "So, it's just us."

Her mauve-colored lips curled up into a smile. "How much longer do you have to keep doing this?"

"Thankfully, this is my seventh round. I only need one more, then a month of Rituxan," I said, with enthusiasm. "I can finally see the light at the end of the tunnel. Oh. That sounded kinda bad. You know what I mean."

"Yes, I do. The tunnel of completing a hard road. Good for you." She gave me a delighted look and then studied me. "If you don't mind me asking, how do you think you got this?"

"They can never tell you why." I rolled my eyes. "It could be any number of things. That's one thing they never have an answer for." [25]

"Oh, I know that." Her hand brushed the air. "No, I'm not asking what they think the cause is. What do *you* think caused it?"

Her question took my breath away. "Uh...." I began analyzing the possible culprits. "I used to drink a lot of diet soda, but I don't do that anymore."

"I didn't mean to be intrusive." She repositioned herself on the recliner. "I was a legal secretary, so I have an interrogating mind." She laughed.

"No, really it's a good question." I paused and gazed absently at a metal tray for a few seconds. Then, it was as if a light bulb suddenly illuminated the answer. "I think stress had a lot to do with it," I said.

"That would make sense. I believe the same for me," she said, her voice relaxed.

Ten minutes later, Nurse Rebecca unhooked me. I said goodbye to my friend and left the chemo room, stopping at a bulletin board in the hallway. I looked at photos of past cancer patients and felt melancholy. I wondered if they were still alive. *Someday, someone has to find a cure.*

It was a chilly December evening. After applying a light shade of red lipstick in our bathroom, I went downstairs, hearing Skylar's voice in the kitchen. I was excited, wondering what he would think of the short, dark wig I'd saved to wear at my work Christmas party. I pondered how long it would take my co-workers to recognize me.

I stood at the base of the steps, feeling sentimental, admiring the framed photos on the family room wall that I took in Spain and Portugal.

Skylar walked up behind me. "Babe, you look hot," he said, wrapping his arms around my waist. He kissed my neck; his cologne smelled inviting.

I turned toward him. His strong facial features and mellow confidence excited me.

"At least I won't be hot during the party," I said, smiling coyly at him. "The medicine's made my hot flashes disappear."

We released our embrace, and he adjusted his loose gray shirt while looking me up and down. "I love this wig on you," he said, seduction in his eyes.

"How lucky are you?" I chuckled. "You have three women for the price of one." I kissed him lightly and put on my leather jacket as he grabbed the car keys.

We'd been getting along well and had hosted Thanksgiving at our house with my family, his kids and family, and a few friends. It seemed to deepen our bond.

We drove twenty minutes up the coast, passing charming beach towns with their own unique characters. "Silent Night" played on the radio. We passed shops and houses decorated with Christmas trees and colorful lights, putting me in a joyful mood.

"Ya know, I don't miss working holidays," I said, petting Skylar's hair. "I can't count how many I've worked."

"Us normal people have holidays off," he said with a grin. "Maybe someday you'll want a job with better hours."

"And miss the twelve-hour excitement of the ER? I'm not ready for that."

We arrived at the Tale of the Whale restaurant, overlooking a scenic bay. I held Skylar's hand as we walked in, happy the uncomfortable times between us had flittered away. The restaurant's large windows opened to views of boats ornately decorated with Christmas lights. They paraded by with people partying on deck. Colored lights twinkled off rippling water.

I kissed Skylar before entering the party room. I felt close to him, my rock through the tough times.

Sounds of conversation and laughter bubbled up from the more than two-hundred people. Overhead Christmas music was barely audible. White tablecloths covered the tables, and cushioned chairs were positioned in the periphery of the square room. A wooden dance floor in the center was filled with people mingling.

I exuded confidence wearing my dark wig, black outfit, and sexy heels. Skylar held my hand, then let go and stepped back when hordes of my co-workers surrounded me.

"Oh my gosh!" exclaimed Cassie, the ER tech who'd given me a journal. "You look wonderful." She wore a hippie-looking long charcoal skirt and green blouse.

"Thanks," I said, hugging her, grateful for the compassion she'd shown me during treatment. She told me she and another co-worker had prayed for me on one of their breaks.

Five nurses wearing cocktail dresses lined up to hug me. "You look sexy in short, dark hair," one nurse said. I beamed; again they made me feel like a movie star.

The next hour was filled with my boss, doctors, ER techs, nurses, and other co-workers swarming me with affection and hugs. I felt happy among them.

Dr. Biden, a bald surfer-looking doctor, ran toward me. "Look at you, Miss Fabulous." He gave me a deep hug. "How are you feeling?"

"I'm great. Thankfully my final chemo is next week, and then I need a month of Rituxan. Then I'll be done!"

"Good." His blond eyelashes accented his light brown eyes. "I want you to know, you're my favorite nurse to work with."

"Aww." *Bashful me.* "Everyone's making me feel so special, like I've just been crowned prom queen."

"Well, then you need to have your dance."

He escorted me to the dance floor, where some nurses joined us. The DJ was spinning top-forty songs, and the floor hummed with bodies shaking to the beat. The mirrored disco ball rotated, casting light around the room. We danced and laughed in a big circle. Out of the corner of my eye I spotted Skylar sitting at a table, looking content.

I danced three songs, and then felt tired. I walked to Skylar and sat on his lap. Wrapping my arms around his neck, I looked into his eyes. "I want to dance one more song – with you."

A slow song played; "I'll be There" by Mariah Carey. He gently escorted me to the dance floor. We danced close.

"I love seeing you happy," he whispered in my ear.

I kissed him tenderly, feeling relief in my soul. My life was turning back around.

Weeks later, I approached the cancer center for my eighth and final CHOP treatment as droplets formed on the manicured shrubs, I inhaled the scent of rain, soothed and calmed. With scars from my cancer battle etched into my soul, I entered the chemo room. The arduous road had come to an end. *Finally.*

Nurse Rebecca escorted me to a recliner. This time, the freezing coldness of the chemo room didn't irritate me. I was in an upbeat mood. She wore a printed scrub top with big pockets and had dyed her short hair strawberry blond. I liked it and thought, *new hair, new year approaching.* She handed me a Benadryl. I gulped it down.

"The final round, Christine. How do you feel?" she asked with a softness I hadn't heard from her before.

"I'm so ready," I said with enthusiasm. "What a road."

"Now you can see the finish line." She gave a likeable smile then left the room, humming a Christmas tune.

She returned with supplies to access my port.

"You're in a happy mood," I said, enjoying seeing her that way. "And I love your hair. New beau in your life?"

She blushed and said, "Let's just say things in my life have taken an upswing."

"I'm glad for you," I said, delighted her road, as well as mine, was appearing better than before.

As she inserted the needle and hooked up my IV, I looked at the three other patients in the room. I guessed they were newly diagnosed because they had hair and I'd never seen them before. I was glad they looked relaxed. Sometimes knowing too much is a bad thing. I smiled at each of them, and then closed my eyes, sleepy from the Benadryl. I thanked God I could see the top of the mountain.

An hour later, my Rituxan treatment complete, I awoke to Nurse Rebecca taking my blood pressure. I scanned the room and saw a bulletin board plastered with Christmas cards. Dangling from one edge of the board was a bronze medal.

She hung a red IV bag and connected it to my line.

"What's the deal with the medal over there?" I asked.

"One of Dr. M's patients ran a marathon and gave him the medal."

"That's really cool." I thought, *whoever finishes chemo deserves a medal. So does Dr. Mahdavi.*

Two hours later, my chemo was done. Nurse Rebecca took down the tubing with her Smurf blue gloves. "You're at the finale, except for four weeks of Rituxan." Her mood changed to motherly. "Oh, and don't forget you need scans after that."

"I know," I said, shaking off her negativity. "Yay! I'm so happy!" I smiled so widely it hurt. "The Rituxan's no biggie. Getting through the chemo was my marathon."

She removed the needle and I stood up. I eyed the other patients and said, "You can do it." I wanted to be their cheerleader.

A sixty-something gentleman with a crew cut gave me a nod and a hesitant smile.

Nurse Rebecca met me in the hall. "Congratulations." I was surprised how cheerful she was, enveloping me in a warm hug.

I put one arm around her and reciprocated. I understood where Nurse Rebecca was coming from. She needed to keep the trauma of what she dealt with all day in the borders of her mind and heart, not spilling over into her job. She cared. She just had to function in the midst of the intensity. She needed to be clear-headed, keeping the sorrow at bay. I thought about how I used to process the way I dealt with people in tragedy. I too, tended to digest the day in my own thoughts. I didn't talk much with friends and family about the sad cases. I had learned to keep the distress in the confines of my mind and heart. That's why my patients' insights and their souls are deeply embedded into mine.

She released from our embrace. "Come with me," she said in her usual detached voice.

She escorted me to Dr. Mahdavi. He sat at a makeshift laminate desk in front of a computer. He looked tired, deep bags under his brown eyes. He stroked his moustache.

"What's up?" I asked, feeling compassion for him.

"I have a new-diagnosis non-Hodgkin lymphoma patient who I'd like to have receive CHOP and Rituxan on the same day, like we did with you." He had a clinical expression on his face. "Can you talk to him about how you liked having both on the same day?"

"Sure!" I felt as if we were back to our doctor-nurse relationship. I chuckled, liking this familiar feeling. Just like the hospital, there was no time to pause for a celebratory moment. Life, and the business of being in the medical profession, goes on. This I understood. Things weren't all about me; I was there to help others on their journeys.

I spoke with the forty-something male patient. He asked me questions and, like the nurse I was, I poured answers and compassion toward him. It was an honor to help. I knew then that in the future a huge goal of mine would be to assist cancer patients as much as I possibly could.

As I walked out of the office and down the elevator to the front lobby of the cancer center, my heart beat quickly. I heard the automatic doors close behind me, and stepped onto wet asphalt, feeling the spatter of raindrops. I lifted my head and arms to the sky. I was overjoyed.

Like an enthusiastic child with news to share, I ran out to Skylar, who waited in the car. I saw him through the windshield and smiled widely, giving him a thumbs-up. I pulled open the passenger's door and leaped into the seat. "I'm done with chemo!" I beamed with excitement. "Minus one month of Rituxan, but that's no biggie." I took a cleansing breath. "I'm so happy!"

"That's fantastic."

He hugged me tight for a couple minutes. I heard him choke up with tears. All I could do was smile and hug him. I felt as if my heart were going to burst.

"I can't even express to you how ecstatic I am." I sat with one knee on my seat facing him. "Thank you so much for helping me through this." I teared up.

"Babe, I wanted to be there." He held my face and kissed my tears. "You mean the world to me."

When we started our drive to the house, the light rain stopped and gray clouds opened to a partially blue sky. I didn't pay attention to the stop-and-go traffic on the ride home. As if I was a teenager, I dialed the phone and talked non-stop to everyone I knew. I called my sister and mom. Each was elated, relief obvious in their voices. Feeling as if I couldn't get any happier, my mom handed the phone to my dad.

"I'm done with chemo!" I practically sang the words.

Silence on the line. I paused and listened to his quivering masculine voice say, "I'm so thrilled."

He began to sob. My heart ached for him. From a man who I'd only heard cry one other time in my life, this experience had brought him to the deepest parts of fatherly love.

"You're making me cry." I laughed and cried in the phone. If anyone understood trauma and a life-changing event, it was my dad. His head-on collision, twenty years before, had brought him near death's door. While hospitalized for three months, he was connected to many machines and tubes, and endured countless hours of physical therapy. His incredible will to live pushed him through, as well as all the prayers sent his way.

I hung up the phone and felt the deepest aching thankfulness I'd ever known. I was on cloud nine.

The next morning, I blinked, pulled the down comforter close to my neck, and stared at the corners of the ceiling, assessing how I felt. I swallowed, noticing I had no bitter taste in the back of my mouth and no nausea. Hesitantly, I stood up and walked to the spare bedroom, still concerned that nausea could grip me anytime. I opened the blinds, curious to see how the day was going to play out.

Droplets of water beaded the lawn, making it look lime green. Trees were heavy with dew. Dark clouds hovered in the nearby sky, spilling sheets of rain. I felt the sun's warmth, and saw its rays penetrating the clouds.

I looked toward the neighbor's house, and spotted colorful arches of a double rainbow. I blinked hard and perched myself on the bed next to the window. Leaning my elbows on the windowsill, I looked at it again, thinking how rare it was to see rainbows in Southern California, let alone double rainbows. The emotions of the past months swelled inside me, and I cried. Nature's beauty was blessing me this day. I felt in awe of this gift and promise of better times to come. I wiped tears from my face, and inhaled a cleansing breath. *Thank you, God.* There had to be a reason for all I'd gone through. I was confident my life was being guided for something bigger.

Chapter 22

Out of the Blue

Thick fog blanketed a beginning of January late morning. Having completed a Rituxan treatment, I sat in one of Dr. Mahdavi's patient rooms, a little groggy. I was glad that was my only side-effect compared with the nausea monster after chemo. I counted down the days, only three more weeks of Rituxan treatments, while waiting for Dr. Mahdavi. I wondered when I'd be able to return to work. I gazed at the familiar framed world map with its many colorful countries, excited to think about my next travels once I was healed and my work schedule allowed.

The door opened. Dr. Mahdavi came in and sat on a metal-based stool.

"How's your day?" I asked.

His moustache stretched into a grin. "Very good."

"My six-month leave from work is almost up, so I need to let them know when I can go back." I felt a sense of relief knowing my entry back into normal life was around the corner.

"Oh." He paused. "Let me give this some thought." He opened my manila-colored chart and reviewed notes. "Considering you're going back to the ER with all the possible germs imaginable, I want you to be off until the end of March."

My eyes grew wide with shock. "What? What...if I just go back per diem and work...a couple days a month?"

"Your immune system needs to build up, and I want to make absolutely sure it's at its best before you return to that environment."

I allowed the news to settle into my mind. "Okay."

For the past month, I had felt ambivalent and fearful about going back to the ER. Did I want to deal with that much stress? Could I keep up with the fast pace? Was that where I was supposed to be after having cancer? My thoughts bounced back and forth.

Then anxiety took its hold: my voice raised an octave. "My boss said they're holding my job as long as possible, but I know they need to hire other nurses. Being on leave keeps my position frozen." I swallowed hard. "Of course, there's no doubt I want to be safe, and I do need to build my strength back." I scratched the new stubble on my scalp through my wig. "I just need a note to give my boss."

"Not a problem." He scooped up the chart. "Settle your mind. It's a new year filled with possibilities."

He smiled and gave me his calm fatherly look and then left the room, shutting the door behind him.

I shook my foot, my legs crossed. I caught myself slouching and straightened to sit tall. Unsettled, I folded my hands, bowed my head, and prayed. I wanted a new year filled with health and my life moving in a positive direction. I took a cleansing breath. I finished my prayer, and stood in front of the world map. Closing my eyes, I pointed my finger and circled my hand in front of the map, and then placed my finger on it.

I opened my eyes. I was pointing at China. "Uh..." Disappointing. I really wanted to go to Argentina.

I removed my finger, reminding myself that it was doubtful I'd travel any time soon. That deflated me. I felt the hints and plans of re-entering what used to be my normal life still lay distant. As my hope teetered, I wondered if this year was going to include uncertainty and a continued bumpy roller-coaster ride.

The next morning, wrapped in my comfortable robe and fuzzy socks, I sprawled out on the living room couch and watched *Seinfeld* re-runs, my feet elevated on a stiff pillow. I'd slept eleven hours, but still felt tired. Through my cancer journey, I'd slowly learned to put guilt aside in all its forms – guilt about sleeping too much, and guilt about dragging down my loved ones. I now listened to my body and did what it asked, unlike before when I'd always push myself to extremes. Restful healing was the best I could offer it.

I lifted my leg toward the ceiling and felt its stiffness. I attempted to grab my foot with my hand, but could only reach my ankle. Irritated, I stood up and did a forward bend, trying to touch my toes like I used to. My muscles were tight. My back cracked. With fingers dangling, I could only reach my lower calf. I raised the cuffs of my pajama bottoms to find scrawny legs with no muscle tone. Frustrated, I took off my robe and hoisted up my pajama sleeves, revealing a pair of bony arms.

I flung my robe over my arm and marched upstairs. I needed to start getting back in shape.

At a women's gym, I signed up and got the schedule for yoga classes. Mirrors decorated the walls. Exercise mats and racks of barbells sat against a side wall. A few women pedaled exercise bikes. I placed a thick royal blue mat on the floor and sat Indian-style, watching my workout in the mirror. I lifted one arm up, bent my elbow, and pushed my bent arm toward my back. My muscles were stiff and taut. I raised both arms and stretched toward the ceiling. Taking a deep breath, I challenged myself and kept them up for ten seconds. I lowered my arms, fatigued, curled my hands in my lap, and gazed into the mirror. I gave myself a mental pep talk.

I reclined on the mat and stretched my body as if someone were pulling me with a rope at opposite ends. It felt good. This whole process had been a tearing down at every level. Building my strength and stamina would be an escalating road of time, hard work, and patience.

In spite of the drizzly, cold, mid-January afternoon, I took a walk around the neighborhood. I pulled off the scarf around my neck, warm after challenging myself with a faster stride. Before entering the house, I rubbed my tennis shoes on the plastic mat.

The house was quiet. Skylar wasn't home. *Good.* We'd fought the night before about the way he pressured me to look at houses again. I told him I didn't feel comfortable spending money on a new house, especially when I wasn't sure what would happen with my job. He ended the evening getting drunk again. It made me disgusted and irritated. Even in the morning, I still felt the heavy tension between us.

I stripped off my coat and placed it on a chair in the family room. My cell phone rang. I ran to the kitchen counter and answered.

"Hi Christine; it's Dominique."

"Oh hi," I said, suddenly focused. A burst of energy hit me. "What's up?" I forced enthusiasm, knowing my ER job was hanging on her words.

"Remember how I told you last week I couldn't guarantee we'd be able to extend your leave?"

"Yes..." My heart pattered rapidly.

"Well, I really tried. HR won't let me hire another nurse with your position on hold. They won't extend your leave, and I know you can't come back to work right now." She took a breath. "I can't hold your position for that long."

I felt a lump in my throat and cleared it. She sounded sympathetic. With the most confident voice I could muster, I said, "I understand."

"I did all I could," she said sadly. "I absolutely want to make sure you know the ER definitely wants you back. Please don't take it personally."

"I know there are rules," I said, grief and resolve in my voice. "It's a business like anywhere else."

"Really Christine, I feel so bad about this."

"I only have kind thoughts toward you and everyone. You've all been so amazing to me."

"You're a special lady. I love you," she said tenderly. "I'll let you know what things need to be done next."

We hung up. I placed the phone on the counter, and sat on the living room couch, pulling my knees to my chest. I peered out the sliding glass door window, where large puddles of raindrops pooled on the concrete patio. It surprised me to feel relieved and scared at the same time. Still, the door had been shut. My ER career was over. *Now what am I supposed to do?*

The image of a giant anthill came to mind. I saw myself piling more loss and change to the list.

A few days later, I hovered over an opened newspaper on the coffee table, enjoying the morning sunshine filtering in. Skylar was making pancakes for his kids, who had spent the night, and for me. He whistled with a carefree attitude, appearing to have no remnants from his drinking binge the night before. I tried not to think about the long-term effects his regular misuse of alcohol might be taking on his body.

Instead, I felt a peaceful determination to search for a new job. "It's funny; I've never looked for a job in the paper before," I said to Skylar, who was standing over the griddle.

"What'd ya do before?" He wiped beads of sweat from his forehead.

"When I did my final student rotation at the cancer hospital, they asked me if I wanted to work there as a nurse. So I did." While I talked, Skylar handed a plate of pancakes to his son. "Otherwise, I've just gone to the hospital where I wanted to work and applied. Nurses are pretty lucky. It helps there's a nursing shortage."

"So what type of job are you thinking of?" Skylar placed a plate of pancakes on the coffee table.

"I'm not sure, but I'd like to give back and use my newfound knowledge and experience," I laughed, "to somehow help others." I tossed the travel section of the paper aside and picked up the classifieds.

I turned the thin pages to the nursing want ads. I crouched next to the table, leaned my elbows on it, and hovered over the paper.

"Wow! This is weird. This job just popped off the page at me like it was in 3D. I've never had that happen before."

"What does it say?"

"It's for a Bone Marrow Transplant Coordinator position at a children's hospital." I took a sip of orange juice. "I was a bone marrow transplant nurse before, so this is something I know, except for the pediatric part."

"Sounds like that would work."

"I have a weird sense this is the one."

I tore out the ad and closed the paper, energized by my new possibility. Smelling the buttery aroma of pancakes, I took a bite and savored the maple syrup, thankful things tasted the way they should. I chuckled, remembering times I'd hardly been able to eat a chicken strip. Maybe the year would be filled with surprises I didn't expect.

It was the third week of January. I was bundled up in bed when I woke up abruptly at 3:00 a.m., threw off the covers, and raised my leg in the air. I grabbed my foot. "Owww! Oww! Owww! This so pisses me off."

"What's going on?" Skylar asked, groggy.

"I'm having those stupid foot cramps again." I clutched my foot and pulled it toward my head, stretching it back and forth to work out the cramp.

"I thought you started medication for that."

"I just started Neurontin two days ago. It'll take some time to kick in." [26]

I stood and leaned my hands on the side of the bed, stretching my feet as if I were a sprinter warming up before a race. Feeling some relief, I sat and cradled my foot, bending it in flexion and extension movements.

After a couple minutes, the cramp went away.

"So annoying," I said, lying back in bed and snuggling under the covers next to Skylar. "Sorry to wake you."

He turned on his side opposite me and fell back asleep.

I sensed his irritation. I couldn't blame him. As much as I'd begun moving toward a life without illness, I couldn't ignore the reminders my body wasn't fully back to normal. For the last month, I'd sensed people close to me were tired of towing the line. When they asked how I was doing, I'd excitedly rattle off that I was almost done with Rituxan treatments. Even though they'd seen my arduous road, they still dealt with the realities and struggles of their own lives. My exuberance in overcoming my hurdles didn't seem to spark their lives anymore. I felt alone. They didn't get my survivor mentality.

I turned on my back and looked around the room and its different shades of darkness. Staring at the gray ceiling, I felt fearful and uneasy. A barrage of questions swirled in my head. I knew chemo had possible short-term and long-term side effects. *What possible issues will I have in the future? Will I start my period again? Can I have children? Will I regain my energy level?*

Then I came to the worst question of all. *Will it ever come back?*

I began to cry. Anxiety made my heart race. I turned toward the closet mirror and saw the silhouette of my bald head. Sitting up, I took some tissues from the nightstand and dabbed my tears. *Just stop,* I told myself repeatedly. *Don't let fear win. There's nothing I can do about it.*

Inhaling deep breaths, I let out a sigh. I focused my gaze on the closed blinds, and heard the rustling of trees move with the wind. *Whatever you want, God. I can't live like this.*

I pulled the comforter up to my face and smelled its Bounce dryer-sheet scent. I closed my eyes and pictured my hand gesturing to stop. Calmness rushed over me. Worrying wouldn't do me any good. Inhaling again, I felt peace.

One thing cancer had taught me was to be more in tune with God and have Him as the compass for my life. I'd decided that in the future, I'd make a conscious effort to pray more, listen to His guidance, and act on my inner nudgings. I needed to stop and let God figure it out.

Chapter 23

Release

Being a cancer survivor doesn't only mean surviving cancer, it also means surviving the many challenges involved with the cancer journey.

I felt energetic as I stood in the brightly sunlit spare bedroom. I walked to my desk and stuffed my extra resumes into a wooden slot. For me, February no longer would have an emphasis on romance. It was a month of being set free. No more sitting in the chemo room receiving CHOP or Rituxan treatments. I was done.

I'd just gotten home from my interview at the children's hospital. I thought it had gone well, and hoped the director of the oncology unit, who had interviewed me, would call for a second interview. I wanted to organize the scattered papers on top of the desk, another goal for the day. I pulled out the maroon desk chair and sat with crossed ankles. The top of my skirt comfortably touched my stomach, and I was glad for the ten pounds I'd gained. My business suit fit again.

While sorting through papers, I recalled some of the interview and started questioning myself. I wasn't worried about my resume. My oncology and transplant experience spoke for itself, but I did tell the director I'd completed cancer treatment recently. *Maybe I shouldn't have said that. No employer wants to hire a person with a medical issue!* I grew scared. Had I hurt my chances of getting hired? I tried to divert my attention by putting receipts of paid bills into a red folder and opening a drawer. *Well, of any job, especially considering this one involved working with children who had cancer, disclosing this information should add to my value as a nurse.*

I put the folder into a hanging file holder and shut the drawer. *I can't think about what I should or shouldn't have said. I have to let it go.*

I shuffled through more stacks of papers, and was startled to find one with my chemo treatment plan. Instantly, a wave of memories of throwing up came to mind, and I tasted bitterness in my saliva. I pushed back the feeling of wanting to gag. Anger filled me. *When does this crap end?*

I opened the bottom drawer and shoved in the paper face down, slamming the drawer closed. I paced the room, consumed by rage. Throwing my wig off, I yelled at the top of my lungs, "Can't I just fucking move on?"

I restrained myself from throwing the trophies that sat on the dresser. Instead, I walked in circles. I felt a lump in my throat, then plopped on the bed and buried my head into a pillow.

"Ahhh!" I yelled, feeling my face smash into the cotton pillow. I turned my head to the side, and stared at the white wall.

Just when I'm moving on with my life, I get a jarring reminder, pulling me to the past.

Tears clouded my vision, along with overwhelming grief. I cupped my hands, buried my face, and drew my knees to my chest. I bawled like a baby. Immersed in sadness, I shook and cried intensely for twenty minutes.

Hiccups came over me. I slowly got up and walked to the bathroom, fatigued. Grabbing toilet paper, I blew my nose, then walked into the master bedroom and changed into a pair of brown sweats. I headed back into the spare bedroom, lighter from my cathartic release.

I lay on the bed, staring at the desk, the papers organized neatly in slots. *Why am I so emotional, even after I'm done with treatment?*

I inhaled deeply. The hiccups were gone. I'd been awakened to depths of emotions I rarely felt. Through this experience, I was establishing a new camaraderie with my feelings – and, hence, the feelings of my patients.

The top of the desk was stacked with old cards and papers in a pile. Even though it was a mess, I knew I could straighten them out and put them in their rightful places. I was surprised to be reliving the grief. I reflected on past patients I'd taken care of in the BMT unit. It was always a jubilant occasion when they left the hospital after staying, sometimes for months. The nurses sent them off with medications, hugs, and celebratory hearts. Never did I realize what they went through emotionally once they left the hospital. By living with cancer, hidden parts of my heart and soul were awakening through the grief. I was seeing things much differently.

On a rainy Saturday night, one week later, Skylar pulled into an Italian restaurant parking lot and opened the passenger door, holding an open beige umbrella. I got out of the car, wrapped my hand around his on the umbrella, and felt exuberant about my family's celebration of the completion of my treatment. No more chemo, no more Rituxan treatments. It was time to celebrate.

Holding tight to each other's hands, Skylar and I ran toward a restaurant topped with a large green and red neon sign, "Buca di Beppo." Heavy rain spattered off the black asphalt as if it were popcorn popping. I heard every click of my black boots on the ground and felt the weight of my wig slap my shoulders with every bounce. I was excited.

Skylar opened the heavy wooden door and we were greeted with the sound of Italian opera, sung by Pavarotti, reinforcing the joy of being somewhere other than the couch.

"This is gonna be fun," I said. I scanned the thick crowd of people in the entry; some were standing, and some were sitting on antique-looking love seats.

"You deserve to celebrate," he said, looking handsome in his black dress shirt and gray slacks. "We're all overjoyed we don't have to see you sick anymore."

We walked to the wooden podium, where a brunette waitress stood, peering at a map of tables. "I guess my family's not here yet," I said into Skylar's ear.

I peered into the restaurant. Waiters dashed by wearing white outfits and red ties, carrying plates of yummy-smelling, garlic-infused food. Black and white photos of people enjoying pasta filled the walls, along with gaudy Italian wall hangings and colorful pictures of the pope.

Turning toward the entrance, I was amused by people-watching and anxiously waited to see my family.

Five minutes later, the oak door opened. My mom, dad, sister, brother-in-law, and two nieces entered. They pushed through the crowd, their faces glowing with glee. My mom was first to reach me. Her blue eyes sparkled and her short blond hair looked recently styled.

I leaned down and gave her a tight hug. "Congratulations. I'm so glad it's over for you," she said, her voice a sing-song of happiness.

We were escorted to a large wooden booth, the table decorated with a red-and-white-checked tablecloth. I sat on the end, and my seven-year-old niece sat next to me. I pulled her close and kissed the top of her head, inhaling her cherry-scented shampoo. "I'm so glad you're here," I said.

After our embrace, she placed her hands on the table and sat tall. She looked cute in her turquoise sweater and Hello Kitty bracelet. "I'm glad you're not sick anymore, Auntie," she said.

"Me, too." I pulled her in for another hug.

My dad sat across from me. His navy sweater accentuated his tan face. As he spoke, I noticed his left eyebrow rose and the right one remained still. His forehead wore a five-inch scar, a reminder of his accident. "So you had the scans and they're clear?" he asked, with a hint of relief. He had dealt with his own cancer diagnosis-prostate, a few years prior. His treatment was surgical resection.

"Yes. Thank God." I perked up as if I were a lit-up Christmas tree. "My PET and CT scans were normal. Dr. Mahdavi said I'm in complete remission!" I beamed. "But I'm not going to use the word remission. I'm cured."

He leaned his elbows on the table, and the waitress took our orders. "Good, it's done," he said, with a wide smile, which he used sparingly. "Now you've gotta put this shit behind you."

"Yeah, that's one way to put it," I said, laughing. "I feel like I've just been freed from jail."

"You have."

Chatter and laughter filled the table. My sister sat on my side of the bench, toward the wall. She looked comfortable in her rose-printed chiffon top. She raised her wine glass. "Let's do a toast." The adults raised their wine glasses, and the kids raised their plastic cups. "To your health. Thank God you're better."

Skylar sat next to my dad and was the first to clink his glass to mine. He gave me a caring look that reminded me of all the loving times in our relationship. Everyone touched glasses.

"This dinner is an exclamation point to my happiness," I said with delight. "I can't thank you all enough for being so supportive and helpful to me."

Two hours later, our evening ended with dessert, hugs, and goodbyes.

On the ride home, the windshield wipers flung heavy rain as the blades scraped the window. I thought about the fun night. Rear car lights looked fuzzy amidst the sheets of rain pounding the freeway. Feeling introspective, I thought about how I was starting to lose the sense of myself as a sick person, a life I'd lived for seven months. I peered at the passenger's side mirror, touched by sadness while looking at distant red taillights. I didn't know where it came from or why it was there, but I knew I didn't want to forget the details of the life I lived as a cancer patient, and the new insights I'd gained. Nestling deeper into my seat, I closed my eyes. *How do I adjust to regular life again? How do I put this shit behind me?*

Days later, I sat outside the oceanfront cliff-side café, enjoying the mildly cool February breeze. The ocean air and the blue water gave me a lift as I watched white caps churn in the distance. Still feeling high from completing my treatment, I looked forward to my lunch with Tonya. I wanted to feel like my old self again.

Scattered tables were topped with crème-colored umbrellas. I took in their simple beauty, my mind at peace. Hearing the crash of the waves, I looked at the shore and saw a black Labrador playfully frolicking in the water.

"Hi Christine," said Tonya in her calm voice, bending down to hug me. As she stood, her brown poncho elegantly draped her tall body. Her dark hair rested on her shoulders. "This place is so perfect. You always know the great hideaways."

"I guess I still got it," I chuckled.

"You never lost it. You were just temporarily out of commission." She sat in the plastic chair and opened the menu.

"So how's work?" I asked reluctantly. A part of me didn't want to know. It felt strange not being employed anymore.

"Same crazy place." She studied the menu and leaned her elbows on the table. "I'm bummed I wasn't there the day you came in."

"It was weird cleaning out my locker."

I shifted in my seat, noticing the touch of stiffness in my back that had been getting better from exercising more and gaining flexibility. "The bonus was that everyone was so happy to see me. I still got the movie star treatment."

"As you should," she said, in a confirming tone. "I can't tell you how often people ask me about how you're doing." She gave the waitress her order.

"That's so sweet. I also stopped by the PACU that day and saw our old cohorts. I had barely walked through the door when they rushed over to hug me. I almost started crying."

"You have a lot of people who love you, Christine."

"I was surprised when the PACU nurse manager told me I was an inspiration." I sipped my iced tea as words from my friend and spiritual warrior Lorraine crept into my mind: 'You don't know what people will cherish from you.' "I'm still blown away and thankful how wonderful everyone's been to me."

We ate our salads. Seagulls squawked and we watched pelicans dive into the ocean.

"So what are you thinking of doing now?"

"I had a second interview at the children's hospital for a bone marrow transplant coordinator position." The breeze grew stronger and I wrapped my sweater further around me. "I think it went well."

"Look at you," she said, putting her credit card on top of the bill. "You just pick yourself right back up."

I laughed, delighted to feel like my old self again, grateful the sadness and intense feelings had passed. “I’m getting used to normal life again.”

We left the restaurant. We walked to Tonya’s car parked on the street, hugged good-bye, and then I headed to the beach. I took off my shoes and cuffed the bottom of my jeans. The sand felt soft and I got a shiver when the cold ocean water rose over my feet. The call of gulls and feel of the breeze on my face soothed me. I’d walked this beach many times and had always enjoyed its beauty, but today it felt different. I wasn’t thinking about a boyfriend issue, my social calendar, or my hectic work life. I was completely engrossed in the moment.

I walked a foot from the shoreline. Kelp and driftwood intertwined where the tide deposited them. I sat on the sand and watched sandpipers run from the waterline, mesmerized by the lull of the surf. The water retreated, leaving glistening sand in its wake. I loved that the beach always looked different, day to day, moment to moment. Always new things to discover. I glanced at the drifting sun and knew in a few hours it would be setting.

This period of my life was coming to a close. I felt as if I’d driven out of a congested tunnel, with people honking car horns, to an open sunny sky and a beautiful coastal view. Finally, cancer was at arm’s length. I was excited and scared to move into the places my life could now go.

Chapter 24

CHANGE OF FOCUS

I peered out the passenger window of Skylar's SUV. The pansies planted along manicured lawns and sycamore trees with baby leaves welcomed spring vibrantly. We were driving to a house for sale that Skylar had already seen. After much coaxing, I agreed to go house hunting with him, even though I felt hesitant. His endless talk about me investing the money from my condo wore me down. I figured the least I could do was be open to something new and show I was a supportive partner. Maybe a new house would be a new beginning.

We pulled up to a yellow single-story, three-bedroom, three-bath house with white trim. It sat at the end of a cul-de-sac in a suburban neighborhood, with shrubs leading up the walkway. Skylar stopped the car and looked at me with hopeful eyes. "I think you're gonna like it."

We stepped out of the car and met his ex-wife, the realtor, in the driveway. Sarah was a slender, seductive brunette with a wide mouth and pouty lips. She looked ten years younger than her age – forty-nine. I'd met her a handful of times. Each time, I felt twinges of inferiority because of her striking beauty and the way they teased each other with inside jokes.

"You two ready to see this great house?" she asked, with too much enthusiasm. She pulled her Prada sunglasses onto her head and batted her blue eyes. Already, I felt they were ganging up on me.

I wrapped my long black sweater further around my body and stepped onto the glossy tiled entry, the click of my boot heels echoing my steps. The vacant house had high ceilings, standard beige carpet, and pale walls. We toured the small master bedroom, and then walked into two other bedrooms. "These would be great for the kids," Skylar said, leading me out of the bedroom, touching the small of my back. I remained silent, feeling both his verbal and non-verbal pressure.

We walked to the family room, which overlooked the covered cement patio. Stepping outside, I heard the noise of cars and saw ivy cascading down the back fence. "It's a little noisy," I said.

"Some outdoor music can fix that." Skylar shot his ex-wife a look. We gazed at the yellow-spotted lawn, and then walked inside, toward the entryway.

"So think about it and let me know," she said, in a matter-of-fact tone. "The smart move would be to put an offer in as soon as possible, but I know you two need to discuss it."

Thanks for the no-pressure sales tactic.

We got back in the car and pulled away. "Great house," he said. "Whaddya think?"

"I think it's kinda expensive and I'm not thrilled with listening to traffic in the backyard." I crossed my arms, uneasy about the entire day.

"Sarah will be able to get the price down. Babe, think about the investment," he said, now in a begging tone. "It doesn't make sense just to rent and throw our money away." He wrapped his fingers tighter on the steering wheel.

The name *Sarah* sent chills up my spine. As well as irritation. "And why do we need to use her as our realtor?"

"Oh, come on. Are you jealous? Honey, we get the best deal by using her."

He inhaled. "I wish I could afford the down payment right now, but I can't. Ya know, my work hasn't been the greatest, and you have the money for it." He shifted in his seat and let out a deep sigh.

My blood pressure soared. "Why do you keep pressuring me? Can't we talk about doing this financially together?" My heart beat stronger. I hated fighting, and it looked like this conversation was heading that way. "Why can't we move and just rent for a while?"

"Damn it," he said in a raised voice. "Do what makes sense!"

I swallowed hard, keeping my sight forward, the stoplights, pavement, and passing cars a blur. "I just don't feel comfortable committing to a house payment and investing my money."

I looked at his silver and sandy brown hair resting next to the seat back. I reflected on how I liked to run my fingers through it, but had no desire to do that now. Instead, I said, "I don't even have a job right now and I just got out of a big ordeal. Let me get my bearings."

I let out a sigh and rested further into the seat, staring up at the grayish white sky.

He pulled the car into the driveway, opened the door, and said, “It would be nice if when I need help, you were there for me.” He slammed the door.

I slumped down further in the passenger seat, my heart stomped on. *Just as I’m trying to pick up the pieces of one part of my life, another begins to crumble.*

As I returned home from my yoga class, late morning rays of sunshine filtered through the living room sliding glass door, highlighting dust particles floating in the air. I’d had three interviews at the children’s hospital, but over a month had passed without a job offer. I’d never doubted my job qualifications before, but now I was starting to. At least I was into a routine of exercising and taking care of house-cleaning duties.

I studied the sunbeams, finding it odd how the dust particles were only visible in sunlight. Like life, sometimes it’s hard to see things until insight manifests what’s really there. I walked to the sliding glass door and opened it. I stretched my arms high, enjoying the mildly cool air, pleased to be gaining more flexibility and tone. I leaned back, relieved my lower back pain had been gone for a week. Feeling energetic, I wanted to clean.

I headed to the sink and began rinsing dishes and putting them into the dishwasher. Emptying a glass tumbler, I caught a whiff of vodka and recalled how Skylar had drunk four vodka tonics the night before. I hated seeing him get drunk so often ... now, five nights a week. I turned off the water, and opened the cupboard above the refrigerator where Skylar kept the vodka. It was three-quarters empty. I closed the cupboard, remembering I saw the new vodka bottle two nights before when Skylar had unpacked the groceries. A feeling of doom crept into the pit of my stomach, and I made myself walk out the kitchen door into the garage. I opened the recycle bin. My heart fell: many empty vodka bottles. I closed the lid and leaned against the tool bench. My world began to spin.

Dazed, I sank to the floor and hugged my knees. What was I was supposed to do. Should I bring it up? We were already having issues.

My cell phone rang. I scrambled inside to the counter and answered it.

"Christine, this is Susan."

It was the director of the Oncology Unit at the children's hospital.

"Hi, how are you?" I said, trying to reclaim my yoga serenity.

I pictured her in her closet-sized, upholstered office, sitting in her swivel chair with her legs crossed. She had blond, bouncy short hair. Disney figurines cluttered her desk. I guess an employee can get away with that at a children's hospital.

"I'm well," she said. "Listen, I'd like to offer you the bone marrow transplant coordinator position."

My heart leaped with excitement. "Thank you!"

"I know this has been a lengthy interview process," she said in an even tone. "We didn't need to fill the position right away. Would it work for you to start the end of the month?"

I was both thrilled and relieved. "That'd be perfect."

We talked about more job details and then hung up. For a moment, discomfort overcame my elation; once I told Skylar, he'd be on me about buying the house.

I walked onto the patio and sat on a plastic chair. Comfortable from the sun's warmth, my heart sang with joy. I was grateful I could now step back into normal life. I rocked in the chair peacefully until mental hesitation crept in. My mind was better after treatment, but sometimes I had issues with concentrating. Could I really do this job? I'd have to learn a new position at a new hospital. Would I get so wrapped up in work life that I'd forget what I'd been through? I wanted to continue the preciousness of my health and continue being thankful for even the simplest things in life, such as drinking a glass of water.

As a bird carried a branch in his beak to a juniper bush nest, I took some cleansing breaths. Like a war veteran returning home, I felt apprehensive and knew there'd be an adjustment period of finding myself at work again, especially going back into the world of oncology. I smiled, though. *Fear can be a good thing.*[27]

Chapter 25

Gaining Momentum

As my own battlefield injuries were being healed, I headed straight back into battle.

Throughout my first month and a half at the new job, I was diligent in learning my responsibilities but also surprised to learn how much of the job involved paperwork, phone calls, and sitting behind a desk. I'd never realized how much legwork and planning were involved in preparing someone for a BMT. It was interesting seeing another view of the process and comparing it with my years as a bedside nurse on a BMT unit. Maybe over time, I'd adjust to the limited patient contact.

The hospital medical record office emitted stale air which contrasted with the sunny May sky I had left when I walked into the hospital that morning. I longed for a sneak-peak at the afternoon, but with no windows and a drab interior, all I got was the feeling of depression. Flipping through papers, I was annoyed with the frigid air conditioner blowing.

Carrying a clipboard, I walked to a counter near the entrance amidst rows of gray shelves stacked with Manila paper charts. I embraced a stack of charts with my name on them and headed to a cubbyhole-type desk. Like a detective, I searched through a patient's medical record in the computer and chart, making sure I understood the cancer treatment they'd had and their test results.

After two hours of searching, I found the appropriate information, copied papers and jotted down dates of test results on my work-up form. I leaned back in the chair and rubbed my eyes, tired and depleted. I was still getting used to four ten-hour shifts per week and trying to regain my stamina. I peeked at my watch; 3:00 p.m. Grabbing my clipboard, I rushed out of the office and up the stairs to the clinic.

At the top of the stairwell, I felt out of breath. I slowed my breathing and placed my palm on top of my head, making sure my shoulder-length strawberry-blond wig was in place. My body was still regaining its strength. At least I'd started my period again; I was very thankful to be out of menopause. Shuffling through papers on my clipboard, I found the paperwork for a doctor in the clinic to sign.

The oncology clinic waiting room was colorful, with a mural of Dr. Seuss-like animals on the walls. People sat in blue chairs while small children played with wooden toys in the center of the room. I breezed through the room toward the door to the exam rooms.

"Christine," a low-pitched voice called.

I turned and saw Greg, a seventeen-year-old patient I was working up for a transplant. He sat next to his mom. "Hi," I said, surprised. "I thought you guys weren't coming to the clinic till next week." I bent down to hug his mom, Marjorie.

"Greg started having stomach pains so we called, and they told us to come in." Marjorie gave Greg a caring look with her walnut-colored eyes, and she patted him on the arm. Each time I'd seen her she'd worn casual sweats, her frosted hair in a messy up-do. She was in her forties.

"I'm so sorry to hear that," I said, noticing his stubble of platinum surfer-hair.

He stared down at his faded jeans and Vans tennis shoes. He'd been diagnosed and treated for acute myelogenous leukemia five years before, when he was twelve. He had relapsed three months ago, underwent chemo, and now sat in remission. He needed a bone marrow transplant to give him the best odds of the cancer not recurring.

I crouched toward the ground and looked into his pale face and sunken blue eyes. "How are you? You look a little green. Are you nauseous?"

He peered at his knees and nodded. I liked his cute freckled face.

"He took some Zofran before we got here," Marjorie said.

I salivated and tasted bitterness in my mouth, reliving my own chemo-induced experience with nausea. My heart ached for him. "I'll tell the nurses and see if they can get you in sooner," I said, sad he would spend the rest of his senior year of high school dealing with a transplant instead of going to prom. His normal teenage life would be radically interrupted by cancer.[28]

Ten minutes later, after speaking with a nurse about patient Greg and getting the appropriate paperwork signed,

I walked outside the clinic. It felt odd to no longer have the job of giving medications to patients and helping them on the front lines of the cancer combat zone. I headed toward the back entrance of the eight-story hospital tower, smelling a foul odor from the garbage bin I passed. Delivery trucks were lined up, idling at the loading dock, their engines uncomfortably loud. Quickly walking past them, I waved my badge over the badge reader and pushed the metal button to enter the automatic sliding glass door. I knew I had entered a fragile world of children dealing with cancer. Amidst feeling tired and sometimes overwhelmed with my new job, I hoped I could be of use to someone here. Every ounce of my being desired to use my new insights and new cancer perspective to help others.

At the end of the day, I drove home beneath a violet sky that filled the horizon, adding beauty to a boring commute. A stream of cars filled the five-lane freeway, their taillights looking like miniature stop signals. I turned off the radio and stared blankly ahead.

At different times during the day, I'd felt my head spinning because I was overwhelmed with so much talk about cancer. Now I was in a daze and didn't want to listen to anyone's thoughts or opinions. The busy day had been filled with meetings, discussions with families, appointment scheduling, and phone conversations with insurance companies. I just wanted silence, and I hoped I could gather my emotional tranquility before reaching home.

My theme of the day had been cancer. I wasn't complaining. I wanted to jump back in and help others through their trials with the beast. Just six weeks before, however, I'd had my Port-a-Cath removed – the final remnant of my cancer treatment. It was not only a relief but another significant marker in pushing the "sickness" reminders away from me. That event earned a celebratory frozen yogurt. I'd also gotten off the antidepressant medication. Even though my hair was growing, it still looked like a boy's, too short for me not to wear a wig. I'd just extricated cancer from my body, mind and spirit, and now I had to learn to be close to it again for the benefit of others.

A blue monster truck roared past me in the right lane. I glanced at it and then looked to the side of the freeway at an unfinished brick wall. There were no construction workers, but I could see two stacks of just-laid gray bricks, as wide as a bus. On both sides of the area was a completed twenty-foot brick wall. The open area gave a view of rows of houses. I thought if I lived on the other side of that, I'd want a brick wall too.

Continuing my drive, I thought of Greg's dilemma, undergoing more cancer treatment and a transplant. My heart bled for him. It made no sense. How does a teenager handle that? How does anyone handle that? Sadness filled me. I pulled off the off-ramp to my exit and stopped at a stoplight, realizing I needed to let go of my thoughts and feelings of the day.

I passed people walking dogs on tree-lined streets. A golden retriever carried a stick in his mouth, and it made me laugh. I was grateful I was healthy and could participate in normal life again. The image of the brick wall came to mind.

I realized I needed to put up some sort of internal barrier to handle the cancer talk about my patients and have it not invade me too deeply. All I could do was pray for my patients, do my job and share my story if it would help them. I was on the battlefield again. I wasn't going to get shot down.

Settling my thoughts, I took a cleansing breath and felt energized, leaving my patients in God's care.

Just three blocks from home, I yawned, exhausted. I looked forward to eating and going to bed early. Twilight was changing into darkness and the day's thoughts were moving farther from my mind. I was finally able to decompress.

I pulled into the driveway and felt uneasy. I knew Skylar wasn't happy I hadn't invested my money in a new house. Here I sat, looking at the faded brown garage door of the home in which I had recuperated from cancer. I paused and gripped the steering wheel, feeling nervous. Another barrier was being built, one with Skylar. I wasn't sure whether Skylar or I were both building it, or if it was me alone, but a definite wall was growing between us. I felt defensive, wondering if it would permanently divide us – or if it could be knocked down.

I took a cleansing breath, pushed the car garage door opener and heard the squeak of it opening. Flinging my purse over my shoulder, I walked through the messy garage and opened the kitchen door. I heard a woman's giggle and saw our neighbor sitting at the bar, drinking wine with Skylar.

Michelle was a large woman who wore tight low-cut tops, bringing attention to her enormous breasts. Her head was piled with fancy blond curls, and she wore fuchsia-colored lipstick.

Disgusted, my anger came to life. Skylar stood abruptly. "Hi Babe, how's your day?" He slurred his words.

I speared Michelle with a glare and then looked down. "Busy," I said. Plopping my purse on the coffee table, I ignored them and headed to the refrigerator.

After an uncomfortable silence. Skylar asked with hesitancy, "Join us for a glass of wine?"

"No. I just want to eat and go to bed."

I pulled out a tub of cottage cheese and took a dish out of the cabinet. I felt their eyes tracking me.

"I should go," Michelle said in her high-pitched, baby-talk voice. She shifted in her seat, picked up her glass, and sloshed wine on the counter. She and Skylar laughed loudly.

I gave her an annoyed glance. "That'd be good."

Skylar darted an unpleasant look in my direction. Michelle quickly drank her wine and walked toward the front door. "I didn't mean to bother you, Christine, I just wanted to talk to Skylar about Little League. We're thinking of enlisting Tegan." She ambled toward the front door.

"Okay. Sure," I said, waving her away.

Skylar escorted her out, and then came back to the kitchen. "That was rude."

"What the hell?" I demanded in a raised voice. "I come home from a long day at work and all I want to do is eat and go to bed, and here you are drunk with the neighbor."

"It was no big deal. So I talked to her about Little League," he said, looking at me with confusion. I smelled his alcohol breath. "You're jealous?"

"No, I'm not."

"You have nothing to be jealous about. Please." He sat at the bar and patted the seat next to him. "My God, Honey, I have absolutely no interest in her. You're leaps and bounds beyond her."

I let out a sigh and pulled crackers from the pantry. I faced Skylar's direction, but didn't look at him. My fury brewed deeper.

"I think a glass of wine would do you good."

"I work tomorrow," I said, irritated. My heart raced. "Drinking doesn't solve issues."

"What's that supposed to mean?"

"It seems that's how you solve your problems," I said, my voice rising again. I looked deep into his eyes and, through them, his soul. "We talked about this before, but you don't seem to hear me. It bothers me seeing you drunk so often."

Skylar hurled himself out of the chair and paced the room.

I recoiled, feeling bad for what I'd said. I took some deep breaths. "So what did you do today?"

"I made some calls and visited a few clients." He walked to the sliding glass door and peered out. "It's slow out there." He gulped the rest of his wine.

"Why don't you look for another job?" My neck grew hot from my anger. I was tired of his excuses. "You've talked about looking into working with another company for a year."

"Babe, you don't understand. It's like this everywhere. The economy's bad."

The kettle reached its boiling point: I exploded. I kept thinking how Skylar had worked only half days for the last nine months, but complained about not having enough money or work. Ever since I'd moved in with him, I had gladly given him money for the mortgage and living expenses. What disturbed me at my core was that he wasn't trying his hardest to make his situation better. He wasn't trying to be the best he could be.

"Why do things have to be so hard?" I yelled. "I just wanna move on with my life, get married, and have a baby." I paused. "Like normal people."

Skylar sat on the couch and ran his hands through his hair. I stared at the tiled floor. There was silence for what felt like an hour.

He cleared his throat. "Let's just get it all out now. Come sit over here."

I noisily placed my dish in the sink, and sat on the couch facing Skylar, studying his strong chin and short sideburns.

"Babe, I love you, but I'm not gonna change. I like how I live my life. And I don't want another child."

My heart filled with a deep ache. "When we got back together we talked about this. Remember when we were on our trip you said if that's what I wanted, you'd gladly do it."

"Well, I changed my mind." He steepled his fingers.

"So, you lied to me?" A sense of betrayal hit me at my core. I held back my tears.

"If that's what you want to think."

I dashed to the stairs and grabbed the banister, hoisting myself upward, feeling shaky and weak, my emotions were raw. In the deepest parts of my soul, I knew I was done. *How do I recover from this?*

Chapter 26

LETTING GO

It had been two weeks since Skylar and I had had our blow-out. I unloaded my car with cardboard boxes for moving onto the floor of the garage and pushed the garage door button, closing my view of the sunny June evening. I walked into the kitchen and placed my keys on the tile bar. Skylar was looking at the patio through the sliding glass door, one hand in his jeans back pocket while talking on his cell phone. For an instant, anger and disgust flashed through me as I imagined him talking to another woman. He'd always been a charmer.

He ended his call abruptly, swung around to face me and cleared his throat. An uncomfortable silence filled the room. We were now roommates, actually acquaintances, and had been trying to avoid the other since our heated discussion.

"So, packing your bags?" Skylar asked with contempt.

"I just signed a lease on a condo," I said, feeling the thickness of pain in the air.

"Good," he said, combing his fingers through his hair. "Time to move on with life."

The sting of his comment made me flinch and made me dislike him even more. I started to tear up but pushed it back. Looking down at my strappy sandals, I murmured, "It's too bad things had to go this way."

"I got plans now," he said, heading out of the room. "So when are you gonna be out?"

"In two days," I blurted, gathering my emotional fortitude.

He dashed to the closet, pulled out his leather jacket and slammed the front door.

I bent down as if I had been punched in the gut. I was glad he was gone.

One evening, four months later, I peered beyond the patio of my rented condo at an overcast October sky that looked like a lavender blanket. The evening's warm breeze tickled my short wavy curls. I chuckled at the feel of my new hair growth and at the compliments I'd heard at work since I decided not to wear my wig anymore. I thought I looked like a boy, but I didn't care. I'd gotten tired of the itchy scalp and smashed hair caused by my wigs.

My thoughts changed. I clutched my hands together becoming nervous about my first post-break-up get-together with Skylar. He wanted to drop off my mail, but frankly I think we both wanted to talk to each other. I felt that I'd gotten through most of the grieving over losing the relationship but hadn't gotten over missing our friendship. I hoped we could get through our first meeting without too much emotional distress.

I crossed my arms and looked at swaying eucalyptus trees in the neighbor's yard. One thing that still lingered and gnawed at me was my feeling of guilt for ending the relationship, especially after all he had done for me. I recalled a few acquaintances saying, "I can't believe you left Skylar after all he's helped you with." Their comments stung and added to my pain and guilt. *Sometimes it's really hard to do what you know is the right thing.*

I heard a knock on the door and greeted him. We gave each other a light hug.

"Come in," I said.

I sat on the navy love seat and he sat on an adjacent wicker chair in the living room. It felt awkward seeing him, and I sensed we both didn't know what to say.

"Thanks for coming over with my mail," I said.

He looked handsome in his business clothes but had large bags under his eyes.

"How've you been?" he asked in a tender voice.

"Good." I felt the strings of my heart tug toward him. "How 'bout you?"

"Fine. Work is still slow, but I'm okay."

"Listen." I swallowed hard feeling a lump in my throat. "I want to let you know how grateful I am for all you did for me — I couldn't have gone through it without you," I said in earnest. "I can't express how appreciative I am that you helped me through one of the worst times in my life."

He rubbed his chin and rested his elbows on his knees. Looking up at me he said, "I'm glad I did that for you." He paused, and I sensed him holding back emotion. "It made me a better person."

That comment made my heart sing. I'd never wanted to be a burden to Skylar or be a partner who couldn't wholeheartedly sail in the same direction as my future husband. "I'll always have a special place in my heart for you," I said, tearing up. “You are an incredible person. I just think we want different things.”

“It’s okay, Honey,” he said, squeezing my arm.

We changed the subject to our work and families. After fifteen minutes, he said he needed to go. We embraced, holding each other for a few minutes. We missed each other.

I closed the front door and collapsed on my love seat. Emotionally I was exhausted, but I knew I’d done the right thing leaving Skylar. I hoped we could develop a friendship after some time had passed. Now it was too soon and too difficult. Feeling melancholy, I walked outside onto the patio, again noticing the wall of overcast sky in the near distance. I inhaled a deep breath, smelling the aroma of eucalyptus, and gazed at the blue sky overhead.

We now lived in different worlds, with separate lives.

Chapter 27

DISAPPOINTMENTS

Pain is always a teacher.

Fifteen Months Passed

It was a sunny New Year's Day morning. I leaned my elbow on the windowsill and stared out the bedroom window of my roommate's two-bedroom condo, seeing the grandeur of distant mountains sweeping towards a crisp blue sky. Rows of white and beige condos were sprinkled between. I wanted to be happy with a New Year and the beautiful day, but frankly, I was miserable.

My roommate was sprawled out on the living room couch next to my bedroom, watching the Tournament of Roses Parade on television. I'd moved in with her, a friend from the hospital, nine months earlier. I sat on my carpeted bedroom floor, flipping through old photo albums and listening to a marching band play triumphantly, celebrating the New Year. I wanted to celebrate and be glad for the things I'd accomplished in the past year but felt disappointed life hadn't turned out as hoped. I wanted to find a suitable partner and start a life of marriage and family. Instead, I was renting a tiny room, smaller than the one in which I had grown up.

Last night, on New Year's Eve, I'd gone out on a mediocre date that had left me feeling lonely. The sting of how I wanted things to be ached inside me like a gnawing hunger.

Turning the pages of a photo album, I saw photos of Skylar and me in Mexico on New Year's Eve three years ago. We had hugged each other with happy smiles under a scenic archway. The photo and memory filled me with warmth. I enjoyed reliving fun times, and I still missed our togetherness. The ease between us, I realized, wasn't easy to find.

After we broke up, almost eighteen months ago, I'd had a boyfriend for six months, but that had ended. I'd dated other men, but none of them had compared to Skylar or offered what we'd had in our relationship. Was I asking too much? Had things really been that bad in our relationship? Why are relationships so complicated? I was sad it didn't work out and missed our togetherness. He'd been good to me. We'd been so close and had gone through so much.

As my thoughts grew deeper, they plunged into hard-striking guilt. How could I have been so mean to someone who had helped me through one of the worst times in my life? Did he know how much I appreciated him? *I hope he's okay. Maybe I should call him and wish him a happy new year, just to see if he's okay?*

I picked up the phone and dialed. "Hello," he answered in his gruff voice.

"Happy New Year, Skylar. It's Christine."

A few seconds of silence followed.

"I just wanted to call and tell you again how grateful I am for you helping me through that difficult time in my life."

"Okay." He sounded distant.

"Well, I also wanted to see how you're doing."

"Fine," he said, irritation in his voice.

Our conversation felt like pulling teeth. My earlier excitement about talking with him evaporated. I had hoped he would be glad to hear from me. "What have you been up to?"

"I got married," he said in a matter-of-fact tone.

Wow. What a shock! I tried to remain upbeat. "Wow. That's great. I'm happy for you."

"I gotta go." He sounded hurried.

"Okay, I'm ... I'm glad you're doing well."

He hung up.

I lay back on the carpet, stared at pale blue walls, and replayed his words. I felt hollow and sad. Tears filled my eyes. I wanted to retreat deeper inside myself and hide from the wreckage in my life. Skylar had moved on. I took some deep breaths and unexpectedly let out a chuckle. *Life, ya just never know*. After the initial shock, my emptiness changed to a wave of contentment. I wanted him to be okay. It appeared he was.

"Happy New Year!" the television announcer shouted.

I sat up, closed the photo album and stuck it underneath my bed. Time to move on.

Skylar wasn't living in the past, so why should I?

Chapter 28

All Things New

This had been a transformation, a guiding force from one life to another.

The year passed quickly. I had transferred a year and a half ago to the Oncology Intensive Care Unit (OICU) of the children's hospital for more patient contact. Now, at the end of November, I found myself armed with chemotherapy for my eight-year-old patient, Ethan. Wearing a yellow gown and Smurf-blue gloves, I pushed Ethan's hospital room door open carefully and maneuvered a tray filled with saline syringes, a blue pad and alcohol wipes. I held a red bag of chemo, its tubing dangling at my side. I was back at the front lines of the battlefield, working as a bedside nurse.

The year I'd spent as a BMT coordinator was good experience, but I didn't miss it. Now, I was glad to be working more directly with my patients. One thing I'd learned through living with cancer: to listen to God's direction and heed the desire for change.

The hallway was noisy. It was mid-morning and the secretary's intercom beeped with calls from patients. The medical team chatted at a table in the middle of the small ten-bed ward.

I walked into Ethan's room, which was filled with crayon pictures of his favorite action hero on the partial glass wall. I was again ready to fight the beast for others. This time, I held a whole new level of respect for cancer and a determination to fight it, having taken on its vengeance myself.

"Love the pictures of Spider-Man," I said. Ethan's poster-sized pictures showed Spider-Man apparently preparing to spin a web.

Ethan didn't acknowledge me, but stared at a SpongeBob cartoon on television. He was an adorable blond, freckle-faced kid. His dad sat next to his bed. He looked like a preppy businessman in his cobalt-colored V-neck sweater that hugged his long arms. He glanced up from his paperwork and smiled, his tan reading glasses resting on his nose.

I hung the chemo on the IV pole, and set the tray on a bedside table. I peered out the window and saw blue sky. Watching wind-strewn leaves fly past, I had a passing vision of Ethan playing at recess. Too bad it wasn't reality.

"Okay Ethan, I'm gonna look at your lines for a minute." I set the tray on his bed and assembled my supplies. I disconnected his hydration IV and vigorously rubbed the cap of his Hickman catheter with an alcohol pad.[29]

The door opened and Donna, another nurse, walked in wearing navy scrubs. "Okay, mister," she smiled. "Let me see your armband."

She read his medical record number and name, and I double-checked the chemo bag.

"Yep," I announced. I connected the chemo to his line and pushed the IV start button while listening to SpongeBob's high-pitched voice. I smiled, glad Ethan was entertained and

Dad had work to focus on instead of his despondency over Ethan's leukemia diagnosis. I picked up my used supplies and headed out of his room.

Ethan's Dad looked up at me. "It's started?" He wrinkled his brow, drawing attention to his high forehead and short sandy hair.

I nodded and smiled. How heartbreaking, now this was what they had to look forward to: Ethan getting his chemo and having a transplant. Wasn't it crazy what the new norm becomes?

I walked into the utility room, took off my protective gear, and washed my hands in the sink. An image of myself as a chemo patient suddenly came to mind. I thought of Skylar and felt a pang of loneliness, then dismissed it. I missed the comfort of having someone to come home to.

In the medication room, I overheard a few nurses complaining about their schedules and gossiping about another nurse. I remained silent, thinking how trivial their annoyances were compared to my thankfulness that I was no longer throwing up from chemo, and my scans and doctors' visits were all normal. Since I'd started working at the hospital, I sometimes felt like an outsider with my co-workers. I didn't share their everyday frustrations. My perspective had changed on what was important. I saw life from the vantage point of a cancer survivor, which is to say, in terms of gratitude. Smaller issues no longer bothered me as much. I was happy to be off all medications and feeling well. Good health was so precious.

Jolted by the overhead intercom, I heard the secretary say, "Christine?"

"Yes, I'm here."

"704 needs nausea medicine."

A few minutes later, I headed toward my patient Alysha's room, my clogs squeaking on the shiny linoleum floor. Quickly, I rubbed my hands with hand sanitizer and put on a mask before entering her room. With a syringe of anti-nausea medicine in hand, I rushed in, seeing my bald-headed, three-year-old patient throw up yellow liquid into a gold emesis basin. The pale-skinned, blue-eyed girl wailed in between episodes of vomiting. Her thirty-something mother was standing next to the metal-railed crib, scrambling to hold Alysha in one arm and the basin in the other. Alysha flailed her arms and wiggled her body.

"Let me help you," I said, moving over to hold the basin. The aroma of her vomit gave me a flash of nausea. I held my breath and continued assisting her mom.

Two minutes later, her vomiting and crying ceased. Her dark lashes were wet, and her lips pouted sadly. A sudden hiccup attack startled her. Mom sat in a rocking chair and placed Alysha in her lap. She fiddled with the TV remote until we heard a blaring, but familiar, movie soundtrack.

"*Finding Nemo*," I said, in a high voice. "I love this movie."

I connected the syringe of anti-nausea medicine to her macramé-like rope of IV tubes. She had five IV pumps stacked side by side, on top of each other. I programmed the machine and started it.

Alysha quickly became mesmerized by the talking fish and nestled her bald head deeper in her mom's arms. The room was filled with remnants of their home life. Stacks of videos were stuffed into a cabinet, and the walls were plastered with posters of Barney and hand-made pictures of purple fish. A bright purple comforter covered the couch, topped with fluffy pillows. Stuffed animals filled every crevice of the room. It felt cozy.

"You look really tired," I said to Alysha's mom sympathetically.

A weak smile appeared on her face. "It's hard to sleep around here." The mother rocked the chair. "You just never imagine life's gonna be like this."

She turned to the framed photos of herself and her family that were on top a mini refrigerator. Tears filled her eyes.

"I know," I said.

"Do you?"

"I'm a survivor of non-Hodgkin lymphoma," I said. "I was completely shocked when I was diagnosed. I finished my treatment over two years ago. I didn't have a transplant, but I had eight cycles of chemo."

I grabbed some tissues off the bedside table and handed them to her. I kneeled down next to the rocking chair and looked directly into her eyes. I didn't tell all the patients and families my story, only those I thought it would help.

"And now you're healthy?" she asked, hope in her voice.

"Yes. Sometimes I can't believe I went through all that, but now I'm good."

I was filled with sorrow for her. For the last month and a half, she and Alysha had lived in that room. Mom only left to shower, go to the cafeteria for a break, or dash home to deal with a major crisis with her other kids.

I squeezed her shoulder. "I can't even imagine what you're going through with your daughter. It's good to get those feelings out."

She nodded and dabbed her eyes with the tissue.

"You're a strong lady," I said. "Any parent going through this feels overwhelmed."

She rocked and nodded again.

"We're all here to help you through it. I'll be praying for you."

She held her daughter tighter. "Thank you." She gave me a close-lipped smile. "I guess sometimes that's all we can do."

I embraced her with one arm and left the room. I took off my mask, crinkled it up, and threw it in a trashcan. Having cancer as an adult is one thing. Dealing with a child's cancer is another level of the nightmare altogether.

I took a deep breath, and remembered how I got through my own illness. You need a multitude of medicines, loving people, emotional purging, and prayers to get someone through cancer. Exactly what Alysha and her mom needed.

Chapter 29

Many Angles of Art

One Year Later, almost four years after I conquered cancer

The balmy, sea-scented November evening was perfect for a fundraiser in Laguna Beach. Serving both as hostess and planner of a fundraiser for Colin's cancer-related charity, I felt hurried and excited. I made a last-minute check, walking by food and auction-item tables. The Asian art gallery looked spectacular, filled with oil-painted portraits of Tibetan children wearing traditional wool clothing and Asian women gracefully holding umbrellas. I gazed at a bronze Buddhist figure with long earlobes sitting on a shelf, cross-legged in a meditative pose, on one side of the rectangular room. It seemed focused on what was about to occur. I scurried near the glass front door, put on a smile, and greeted guests.

There was one person I hoped to see more than any other: Mike, a guy with whom I'd had a date the week before.

Since Skylar and I had broken up, I'd dated quite a bit. I'd met many men, but they had lacked the quality and integrity of someone I wanted for a marriage partner. I'd grown tired of being alone. Cancer had taught me how delicate life is and to listen to my intuition and God's guidance, which meant to search hard for things I deemed worthwhile. It had also made me realize that I wanted to be close to God and listen to His nudgings and wisdom daily. As I remembered how much people prayed for me during treatment, I decided it was time to implement out-of-the-box thinking and lots of prayers.

I'd met Mike on a blind date through a dating service. I'd been told about his handsome looks, that he worked in business and had an even-tempered personality, but I hadn't seen his picture. We met for a drink and appetizers at a French restaurant. A day after our meeting, he had called, and I invited him to the fundraiser. He had said he might come.

My sister Karen, who helped me prepare for the fundraiser, stood next to me. She wore a white choker necklace that contrasted with her black flowing dress. We watched a petite Asian woman in a silk kimono elegantly glide her hands across a Chinese Guzheng (zither). With finger picks, she plucked the strings gracefully, giving way to the delightful, relaxing sound of a tumbling waterfall.

"Isn't this beautiful?"

"Adds just the perfect touch," she said, as we scanned the crowd, observing people nibble hors d'oeuvres, sip wine, and chat.

The gallery was filled with cheerful guests, many of them friends who'd helped me on my cancer journey. A doctor with whom I worked at the children's hospital, my boss, and many nurses were in attendance. So was Colin. I was a board member for his cancer organization which involved mentoring adolescent and young adult cancer patients. His non-profit group also provided college scholarship funds for survivors. We both had participated in mentoring cancer patients. Our original nurse/patient relationship had changed into friendship, mixed with a deep commitment to ease the struggles of people on their cancer journeys. We both embraced our history and experiences with cancer and used it to help others.

Colin stood at one end of the gallery talking to guests. He had dark curly hair and had regained his athletic football player weight compared to when I'd taken care of him so long ago. He looked in my direction. We caught each other's glance and he gave me a wide smile. My heart swelled with pride of all he'd accomplished since being a young adult with cancer. It amazed me at how our paths had crossed, and were again converging at this momentous event.

"Looking at these paintings," my sister said, shaking me out of my reverie, "makes me want to learn to paint."

"I agree. That's in addition to my list of life things to do," I said, turning to look at a painting of a Tibetan child.

Since having cancer, I felt my priorities change. I desired to see my creativity blossom further. My interest had always been traveling, but now I found an added passion of helping kids with cancer.

We continued our stroll toward the front of the gallery and chatted with guests. I absorbed the fun energy in the room, a combination of exotic art and people with charitable hearts.

Then Mike walked in, handsome in his blue suit and tie, striking with his smile and kind brown eyes. He was six-feet tall and muscularly thin with dark short hair. He wore glasses.

During our date, he had seemed shy at first, but we had ended up talking for hours. I enjoyed his witty sense of humor and that he was a good listener.

"Oh my gosh." I was suddenly nervous and poked my sister with my elbow. "There he is."

I strolled over to the entrance and greeted him. "Hi, I'm so glad you made it." I gave him a loose hug.

"Looks like everyone's having a good time," he said with a shy smile. He signed the guest book and put on a nametag.

"Can I get you a glass of wine?" I asked.

"Sure."

We ambled toward a table in the center of the room. "Christine," I heard a voice call out.

I turned to Mike. "Duty calls. Sorry, but I need to go greet people coming in the door." I frowned. "I'm gonna be a little preoccupied tonight, but bear with me."

"You're the hostess," he said, picking up a glass. "I expect that."

"Enjoy mingling. I'll be back soon."

I felt a surge of anxiety and sped toward the door, where I welcomed arriving guests. Mike walked the perimeter of the gallery and viewed the art and auction items.

I needed to talk shop with my boss and a doctor with whom I worked, telling them about the most recent updates going on with Colin's program. We had implemented it at the children's hospital.

I saw Mike in the distance conversing with an attractive blond. I felt butterflies and couldn't help wondering if she was flirting with him. After ten minutes, I said to my boss, "Excuse me. I invited a date here, and I need to go talk to him."

She gave me a look of surprise, and broke into a smile. "Where is he?"

I motioned toward Mike, who was staring at a painting. "I don't want him to get too bored. It's technically our second date."

"He's cute," she said, folding her arms over her cocktail dress to study him. "Get over there."

The nicely dressed blond woman continued to talk with Mike. As I approached them, I caught his eye. His face lit up.

"Hi," I said to them. "What do you think of the event so far?"

"Nice," he said. We locked eyes. "Definitely a success."

I introduced myself to the woman. She eyeballed people in the distance and after a few seconds drifted away.

"Not to overload you," I said with a smile, "but I want to introduce you to some people."

After chatting for a couple of minutes, we walked toward my sister and a few friends. She ran her critical eye over him and began probing him with questions. I gave her a "don't-do-it" look, but she continued with her interrogation.

"So where did you grow up? Do you have any kids? What's your passion in life?"

He answered her questions without a hint of annoyance.

"Do you go to many art galleries?" she asked him.

"No, but it's good for me to expand my world," he said with a grin. "Now, do you have any curve balls for me?"

We laughed. "Don't even tempt her," I said.

"Let me take a picture of you two." My sister raised her camera.

Mike looked at me with a dimpled smile. We posed for the photo standing close. I embraced the moment.

Hours later, after the fundraiser had ended, my sister and I walked to my car. "He seems like a genuinely nice guy," she said.

"I think so..."

"I was watching him talk to that girl," she said. "When she asked him questions, he just gave one-word answers. He kept looking for you."

"That's comforting."

I drove down the lamp-lit road, happy. I caught a glimpse of the ocean and the moon's glistening reflection on the water. The night had been a convergence of my past and present, my tribulations turned into passion. I hoped Mike would be a promising part of my future.

Chapter 30

FOOTSTEPS

It's one thing having people cheering you on,
yet another to know they've walked in your footsteps.

Six-and-a-half months later, I looked out one of the empty OICU patient rooms at the distant mountain landscape, enjoying peace before what would most likely be a busy day. The hue of a purple tinted sky added vibrancy to the energy I felt inside.

Months earlier, I'd become the charge nurse of the OICU. The unit was quiet compared to the busyness of most days. It was nice for a change. I knew, as all the nurses did, things could change at any time. We shared an unwritten rule not to jinx ourselves. If a co-worker said, "I can't believe how quiet it is," a nurse would give that person a dirty look and a retort of, "Ugh. Don't say that!" Were we superstitious? I hoped nothing lurked on the horizon to jinx us.

I checked equipment in the empty room, making sure it was functional. While looking at the bed made with clean white sheets, a memory of an eleven-year-old patient I'd taken care of the week before came to mind. She was a sweet girl with gorgeous long hair. I remembered her and her parents laughing about a camping trip they'd taken before she was admitted for her bone marrow transplant. Now she was in the

Pediatric Intensive Care Unit (PICU) and needed to be on a ventilator due to complications from her transplant.

A wave of sadness swept over me. It was another reminder how intense and fragile the process of curing cancer is and, unfortunately, the casualties involved. Taking a deep breath, I re-focused on the present, and headed to the nurses' station for the multi-disciplinary team meeting.

The semi-circular unit included ten single-patient rooms, separate enclosed kitchen, medication, and utility rooms. The nurses' station had two long desks, a secretary sitting at one near the intercom and entrance to the unit, the other topped with computers.

I maneuvered the mouse, pulling up patient data while listening to the team discuss each patient's condition and plan. The team consisted of a physician, nurse practitioner, dietician, pharmacist, child life specialist, physical therapist, and nurses.

I jotted information down on a clipboard already filled with patient data I'd received from the night shift, and added details to the conversation as needed. The meetings were intense, sometimes exhausting. As I focused on what an Asian doctor was saying, the secretary came up from behind and handed me a note, startling me.

I opened it. It read, "You have a delivery." I hid it under some paperwork, keeping focused on the discussion, while the intercom buzzed and phones rang in the background.

Two hours later, the team had left except for the nurses, who were working on their charts. My eyes blurred from staring at the computer screen while inputting patient data.

The secretary walked up with a pleased look on her angelic face and handed me a narrow gold box. "Here's your delivery," she said in a sing-song voice.

All eyes were on me. I peeked inside and saw a dozen long-stemmed red roses. My cheeks flushed with pleasure, happy Mike and I had a flowering romance.

"Read the card, Christine," the secretary said, hovering next to me.

Feeling my heart flutter, I opened the miniature-sized envelope. "It's from Mike," I gushed, happy to be reminded that love was in my life.

I displayed the contents of the box to the nurses. Their eyes grew wide, as did their smiles. "That's so romantic," one said.

I felt as if I were in a fairy tale, so elated to be in a relationship with a wonderful, thoughtful man different from anyone I'd ever met. He was more of a serious type compared to my outgoing nature, but we balanced each other out. We deeply cared for, respected, and loved each other. I'd found a special relationship at last.

I closed the box and asked the secretary to take it to the lounge outside the unit. As she disappeared around a corner, I ached to have this token of love around me longer. I hated letting my flowers go, but knew fungal infections could be spread from plants and flowers to patients whose immune systems had been compromised.

One of the nurses interrupted my euphoria. "Christine, line two for you." I snapped back into work mode.

The clinic wanted to admit a new patient to the unit. I wrote the information on my clipboard, hung up, and walked to the empty room. I began preparing for my newly diagnosed non-Hodgkin lymphoma patient. *The same type of cancer I had.*

While setting up the cables with EKG probes, the shock of my own diagnosis came to mind. I imagined how the child and family felt.

Ten minutes later, my nine-year-old patient, Gavin, was wheeled into the unit. He had red hair, looking as if it were cut with a bowl over his head. His blue eyes were large and his skin milky.

He hopped into bed and looked up at the television in an upper corner of the room. "Can I watch TV?" he asked.

I glanced at his mom, who had wavy blond hair and tear-filled eyes. I smiled and said, "Sure, let me just get you tucked in."

It always amazed me how resilient kids were in trying times. I described the gadgets on the bed and the hand-held call light. "Okay, this is how you turn on the TV." He scanned channels and stopped at *Pirates of the Caribbean.*

"Arrhh," I said, and then laughed.

He giggled and turned back to Jack Sparrow's swash-buckling. I gave Mom an empathetic look. She stood with arms crossed, rocking back and forth, her pretty plump face exhausted. Mascara was smudged on her eyelids.

"Just give me a few minutes to do an assessment on him, look at his IV and read the doctor's orders," I said. "Then I'll come back and explain some things to you."

I left the room, and took a deep breath. I knew their lives would be changed from this day forward. I felt a twinge of discomfort and uncertainty, pondering what to say to Mom. I recalled my own mother had told me to "think positive" when I'd been angry about my diagnosis. I didn't blame her. It's hard to know how to comfort someone in crisis. However, I knew *not* to say that.

Upon re-entering Gavin's room, I heard him laughing at Johnny Depp's antics. Mom sat on a miniature couch staring at her steepled fingers. "How ya doin, bud?"

"Good," he said, enjoying the cheeseburger he'd been given.

"I wanna take your mom on a little tour and show her the rest of the unit. Is that okay?"

"Sure."

Mom gave me a look of fear and I nodded. "It's okay; we won't be long."

A child life specialist walked into the room. I was pleased to see her, knowing how all the support from friends, family, and medical staff had helped me.

"Gavin, do you like video games?" she asked.

His gaze focused on her.

She handed him the Nintendo controls, set up the game "Mario Party," and sat down. He looked happy.

I escorted Mom on the tour. I swallowed hard. "I know this is a huge adjustment."

"I'm not leaving my son," she retorted, seeing a parent exit the unit.

"Parents stay here with their kids," I said calmly, hoping I could give her a feeling of support. "We want you to stay." I showed her how to get to the unit from the main elevator. We walked past a sign that read, "Oncology Intensive Care unit." I buzzed the intercom. "Just touch this button and the secretary will let you in."

Annoyed, Mom let out a huff. "This is the last place I ever imagined I'd be," she blurted.

I understood her anger. A memory of myself in the cancer center came to mind. I remembered how enraged I felt while filling out paperwork on which I had to write what type of cancer I had and how long I'd had it. "I'm sure you're feeling a wave of all kinds of emotions right now."

She rolled her eyes. "To say the least," she said in a stinging tone.

We toured the kitchen and then walked to a board filled with photos of patients. "These are some of the patients who've been here," I said. We looked at the photos of smiling children.

Her posture relaxed, and she seemed to let her guard down. "How do people deal with this?"

"The families maneuver through the shock and become stronger." I patted her shoulder.

"I don't know how I'm gonna get used to it," she said, tears trickling down her face.

I escorted her into an empty patient room and we sat down. I handed her a box of tissues. "Just let your feelings out."

"I've never even heard of this disease before." Her voice cracked as it rose. "This is insane." She cried cathartically.

My heart ached deeply for her and her son. I patted her back as she cried. "I don't tell all the parents this unless I think it will help." I paused and listened to her sob. "This might help you."

She quieted.

"I had non-Hodgkin lymphoma four and a half years ago."

A look of shock swept over her face. She focused on me. "What?"

"Yes. I had stage three NHL. I went through chemo, and I'm now fine."

She stared at the tissue she clutched in her hand. Her face muscles lightened and she sat back in her chair. "I can't believe it." She studied my face.

I smiled. "It's true." I explained my symptoms and the shock of receiving the diagnosis.

She dried her tears. "I'd never even met anyone who had non-Hodgkin lymphoma and now you, his nurse, are standing right in front of me." She shook her head. "You had it and are a survivor." She let out a sigh. "I feel so relieved."

"This is why I'm here," I said, embracing her. "I'm here to help you. We're all here to help you."

We chatted a while longer. Finally, she stood and straightened her polyester blouse, combing her fingers through her hair. "I'm obviously the one who's a mess here. Gavin's the strong one."

I took her back to Gavin's room then walked to an empty patient room. Resting my hands on the windowsill, I stared at the blue sky and picturesque mountain range. Overwhelming gratitude and elation filled me; my eyes swelled with tears.

Cancer had recalibrated my life and deepened my perspective; I could relate to others struggling with the disease and felt privileged to work with the bravest kids and parents I'd ever met. The direction of my life had shifted. It all made sense, aligning to a higher purpose.

Chapter 31

BLISS

Fifteen months later, almost six years after I conquered cancer

I sat like a queen on the plush seat of a white 1937 Packard, en route to the place I would be married. People waved at me on the streets of Laguna Beach. The unusual antique car brought attention, even more so with me wearing my white halter wedding dress and veil. The driver honked the horn, its whimsical note adding more enthusiasm to the event, my wedding day.

Overjoyed, I waved back at people strolling the streets outside art galleries and restaurants. It was a picture-perfect late Saturday afternoon in September. A comfortable breeze blew softly in the bright blue sky. There wasn't an ounce of nervousness in me, exactly how I wanted to keep it.

While driving north on the scenic Pacific Coast Highway toward the wedding site, the tuxedoed driver glanced back at me and winked. He tipped his black chauffeur's cap and smiled. "This is your big day. Are ya having fun?"

"This is so amazing. I feel like a movie star."

He grinned. "Just soak it all in."

We drove by a sandy beach filled with volleyball players and sunbathers. I heard the squeal of kids running from the foaming white wash of the surf. Their simple fun delighted me. It was an average beach day for many, but for me, it was one of the most important days of my life.

We meandered up a hill, minutes away from the wedding site at Heisler Park. Then we encountered traffic.

"We have about ten minutes," he said. "Where'd ya like to go?"

I turned my attention away from the pristine ocean, and looked at the red traffic light. Fear began to bubble inside me. "Uhh," I stammered. "Let's drive by some of these old houses." I pointed to the right.

Nervousness hit me like a wave. I was shocked. Even months before the wedding, I'd felt collected. I lifted my cascading bouquet and smelled a white rose. I remembered my florist one week earlier saying, "You're the calmest bride I've ever seen." I was disappointed that feeling had escaped me now.

After taking a deep breath, I peered out the window at charming houses and window boxes filled with flowers. The butterflies continued to flutter inside me. *Why am I nervous?* I'd been through many changes in life, and now I was minutes away from a most wonderful life-changing moment. I had no reservations about marrying Mike. For this decision, and some others, an inner knowledge felt cemented deep inside.

Quiet with anxiety, I held the handle of my bouquet tight. I knew that one day, I would get married at the place we were approaching, a grassy bluff overlooking a rocky shore of the Pacific Ocean. I knew which wedding dress would be mine the minute I saw it, before even trying it on.

After battling through chemo, I'd read the classifieds and the job opportunity to work at the children's hospital jumped off the page at me. I saw those times as God's nudging confirmations on the path I should take and decisions to make. As messy and jumbled as my life had been, things had worked out for the best. What looked like chaos was really part of a bigger plan.

I stared at my bouquet, and took in its white roses with rhinestones in the center. So beautiful. I thought about how God had given me people to offer His wisdom. Tanner, the ER tech with whom I had worked, told me I should write a book, and so had other friends. Lorraine, my spiritual warrior, always said, "God has bigger plans for your life."

"How ya feeling?" the driver asked, leaning back to give me a compassionate smile.

"Surprised I'm a little nervous."

"It'll be great," he said with reassurance.

I nestled deeper into the comfortable seat and thought of Skylar. He was a wonderful man with many great qualities, but I knew after the cancer treatment that he wasn't my long-term partner. It was very difficult to end that relationship, but I believe he was brought into my life to be my angel and help me during my illness. I prayed that I helped him in some way. The common theme in all these scenarios, God had tugged at my heart and mind, and luckily, I'd listened.

The ten minutes passed. The driver guided us to the wedding site. While passing gorgeous houses along a cliff, I looked at my diamond engagement ring. Peace settled over me.

We pulled up to the curb. Overwhelmed with excitement, I arrived at one of the most beautiful places I'd ever seen. Friends and family stood in the midst of a grassy bluff surrounded by palm trees, its fronds gently tossing in the breeze, the ocean below magnificent.

The chauffeur opened the car door. I stepped onto the curb to the cheers of people, their faces full of happiness as they snapped photos of me. Many had walked alongside me on the treacherous path through cancer, offering their comfort and compassion, and now were there to celebrate the love I'd found.

Lorraine walked up to me with an exuberant grin. She embraced me deeply. "You look beautiful."

The crowd split to form an aisle and the flower girl fluttered her hand, gracefully dropping white rose petals on the lawn. The harpist delicately plucked the strings of the harp and played "Canon in D." Beginning my walk down the aisle, I held my father's arm. I felt as if I were dancing. I smiled at guests and surged with exhilaration when Mike and I locked eyes. He was stunningly handsome in his black tux and striped silver and black tie. He beamed with delight and gave me a tender look. My dad escorted me to the front and offered me to Mike. We interlocked hands and gazed lovingly into each other's eyes as the pastor started the ceremony. I'd met my destiny.

Days later, Mike and I were thankful to be on our honeymoon. We stood in our bathing suits in the center of the over-water bungalow, suspended on poles above the warm waters in Moorea. We looked through the glass-covered hole in the floor and saw an assortment of rainbow-colored fish darting in and out of coral.

"Look how beautiful they are." I crouched down to get a better look. "Let's go out and snorkel off the deck."

"I'll lie on the lounge chair and watch you," he said with a yawn, stretching his arms.

I hugged him around his bare waist. "You gotta go in. They say it feels like bath water."

I took two snorkels out of the wicker basket by the sliding glass door and enjoyed a whiff of plumeria from the tropical bouquet on the coffee table.

Mike followed me out to the wooden deck and relaxed in a lounge chair. I inhaled the salty air and gazed at the turquoise water against its backdrop of lush, dramatic mountains. "This water is amazing," I said, seeing the white sandy bottom and feeling the warm water on my toes. I knew Mike wasn't much of a water person, one of our many differences. He was comfortable with activities on land.

"Look, there's a puffer fish." I put the mask on my face and stepped into the chest-high water. It felt smooth and silky and I could see my feet. "It's so clear."

Five minutes later, Mike moved to the edge of the lounge chair and watched me. He grabbed his snorkel and headed into the water. In his usual way, he said nothing for a couple of minutes, and then swam closer to a neon pink wrasse and raccoon butterfly fish.

Swimming next to him, I reached for his hand. We stood, took off our snorkels, and hugged each other. "Can you believe we're here?" I asked.

"I have to say this is incredible." We kissed, my passion surfacing.

After snorkeling together for half an hour, we climbed the steps to the deck to lie in our lounge chairs. Feeling the seawater dry on my skin, I baked comfortably in the sun. The sun seemed brighter here. Everything seemed clearer, as if I was viewing things through a microscope. I relaxed more deeply into the cushion of the lounge chair and felt the utmost of peace.

Mike and I were good for each other. We challenged each other and supported each other's dreams. I didn't know if our lives would include having children or not. What I did know was whatever happened, I'd be thankful and content.

A sudden image of me lying inside the claustrophobic PET scan machine popped into my mind. I stiffened. Allowing the tension to release, I inhaled a cleansing breath, remembering I'd mentally escaped to Tahiti when I needed to find my happy place – the place I'd wanted to go on my honeymoon.

I watched the lull of the tranquil water in our French Polynesian lagoon and smiled. It had been a long road, but I'd reached my paradise.

EPILOGUE

"Dad, let me help you put your oxygen back on," I said, gently wrapping the plastic oxygen tube behind his ears.

"Okay, sweetie," he said, tiredness in his voice.

The macho man I'd always known now had difficulty standing and needed help walking to the bathroom.

Since I've written this book, my dad was diagnosed with metastatic bone cancer which originated in the prostate. When I heard the news, my greatest and constant prayer for him was for the best outcome. I had the privilege and honor of taking care of him. He gave me the gift of helping him in the midst of his pain and suffering; a true place of vulnerability and trust. It was a chaotic time, but also a time of deep intimacy in our relationship. A sacred place to be and the only place I wanted to be. I was used to playing the role of nurse, my second nature, but hard to be losing someone I loved so dearly. As he grew weaker, he was confined to a hospital bed at home and couldn't move his legs. Turning him, and moistening his mouth with a toothete sponge felt natural. I'd done that with so many patients. Standing at his bedside, I knew my decision to become a nurse was exactly what I should have done.

The day he died, two months after his diagnosis, our family (my mom, sister, brother-in-law, nieces, a neighbor who is like family) and I stood holding hands praying over him in his hospital bed in the middle of the living room. In the midst of the sadness, intense joy and serenity saturated my heart. The energy in the room was actually jovial and illuminated with tranquility. Five minutes later he passed away very peacefully. We had prayed him home. It was beautiful.

A few days earlier, a pastor from church, who was also a cancer survivor, had spoken to my dad about inviting Jesus into his heart. Prior to his diagnosis, my dad hadn't been the most spiritual type. During his final cancer battle, I saw him question his eternity and wonder what's next. That day he decided to pray the prayer of forgiveness. Instead of complaining about his circumstances, he embraced his situation with humor. He called the living room where he lay in a hospital bed, with television clicker in hand, his "Man Cave." A sense of peace permeated his essence. His earthly shackles of sin, disease, and pain evaporated. He was heaven-bound.

I now have another bedside experience and viewpoint, a deeper appreciation and awareness of the difficulty and godliness in the sacred service of being a family caregiver.

God has brought me many blessings, beyond what I ever imagined. I am grateful for being healthy and for being a cancer survivor for over twelve years.

My husband and I never had any children. The child I bore you are reading.

Unfortunately, the world is still battling cancer.
I won't stop trying to be a beacon of hope for those dealing with the beast.

ACKNOWLEDGEMENTS:

Just as it took a multitude of people to help me through cancer, it also took a multitude of people to help me with this book. I am extremely grateful for both sets of people.

There are many individuals to thank:

Immense gratitude I pour out to Dr. Mahdavi, Dr. Kroll and to all my nurses, doctors and co-workers! You live the life of a nurturer daily and it means so much!

Janet Simcic, for pointing me in the right direction in the book-writing process. Thank you for being a mentor, guide, and friend.

Louella Nelson, my mentor and instructor. Thank you for your wisdom, constructive feedback, and diligence in helping your students. Thank you for honing my writing skills.

Members of my writing group: Judith Whitmore, Dennis Phinney, Wally Runnels, Dennis Copelan, Will Hager, Cynthia Slocum, Michele Khoury, Colleen Dempsey. Your honesty and feedback helped me greatly.

Special thanks to Paula Henry, healthcare attorney, for your expertise and advice regarding legal matters for this book.

Elaine English, literary attorney, for helping me with contract paperwork.

Writing a book is definitely a lesson in patience and refining. Special thanks to the following individuals who helped with editing at different stages of this book: Kristin Lindstrom, Robert Yehling, Inga Neubert, and Langtons International Agency.

Inga, thank you for your editing talent. I cherish our extraordinary friendship and have it tucked inside my heart in a special place.

Corinne Gronnel, thank you for creating the Nurse Talk icon and book cover. You are an insanely talented and wonderful friend. Your creativity is contagious.

To my family, and friends who are family. You are in my heart always. I appreciate all the help and encouragement you gave me throughout my treatment and with this writing endeavor. I inhaled your support.

Karen and Andy, through tumultuous times to times of celebration, thank you for being there.

To my nieces, Taylor and Alyssa, thank you for your beautiful, healing energy and enthusiasm about life and about this book. I am so proud of both of you.

Mom, you always said, even when I was young, that I would write a book. Thank you for believing in me always, loving me always, and supporting and encouraging me down every path I have forged. God has filled your heart with huge love. I am grateful that you are my mother.

Dad, you always asked, "When is your book going to be done?" The book-writing process was a long road. I feel your heavenly support and encouragement. Thank you.

A special belly-rub thanks to my constant canine companion, my Schnauzer. You kept me company during the long, lonely hours of writing this book. You nourished my soul in your own furry way.

And, my incredible husband Mike. I could not have accomplished this goal without your endless love, support, and patience. You are truly a gift from God and the most amazing man! My life is beyond blessed because you are in it. Thank you from the bottom of my heart!

Ultimately, I thank God for making my life an incredible journey.

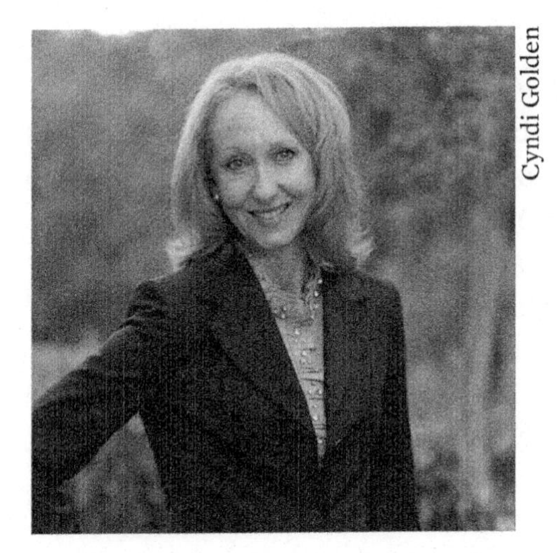

Cyndi Golden

About the Author

Christine Magnus Moore, RN, BSN, has spent fourteen years as an oncology nurse for adults and children and obtained a Master's Certification in Caring for Teenagers and Young Adults with Cancer. She is a non-Hodgkin lymphoma cancer survivor for over twelve years and is passionate about mentoring and helping people battling the beast. Christine currently serves as a Board Member for the Leukemia & Lymphoma Society and is the Chairperson of a young adult cancer survivor group called LLS SoCal Cancer Connection. Wanting others to feel comfort and love similar to what she received during her cancer struggle, Christine cofounded a cancer comfort non-profit organization called YANA (You Are Not Alone)(www.yana-cancercomfort.com) and currently serves as a Board Member.

In addition to writing *Both Sides of the Bedside,* Christine has published articles for the Clinical Journal of Oncology Nursing, the I Had Cancer website (www.ihadcancer.com) and writes her own blog (www.bothsidesofthebedside.com/blog).

She lives with her husband and bundle of fur, a Schnauzer, in Orange County, California.

Please contact Christine through her website at Christine@bothsidesofthebedside.com

Nurse Talk and References

1. Testicular cancer is usually diagnosed in young men and may develop in one or both testicles. Treatment involves surgery, and may require chemotherapy and/or radiation.

   American Cancer Society. (2013). *Testicular Cancer.* Retrieved August 17, 2013, from http://www.cancer.org/cancer/testicularcancer.

2. Non-Hodgkin lymphoma is a cancer of the lymph nodes. Lymph nodes are located throughout the body and act as a filter for the blood to take out hazardous bacteria and particles from the system. According to 2013 American Cancer Society statistics, it is the seventh most common cancer in men and sixth most common in women throughout the United States, excluding basal cell and squamous cell skin cancers. It is a life-threatening cancer.

American Cancer Society. (2013). *Non-Hodgkin Lymphoma facts*. Retrieved May 2, 2013, from http://www.cancer.org/research/cancerfactstatistics

3. Leukemia is a cancer of the white blood cells/bone marrow (where white blood cells are produced) and occurs when there is an overgrowth of immature white blood cells called blasts. Patients receive chemotherapy to put them into remission and, in some cases, require a bone marrow transplant (BMT) for treatment. Following a bone marrow transplant, patients receive daily lab work to assess if their bodies are accepting the donor's marrow as its own, demonstrated by making new white blood cells, a process called engraftment.

4. Prior to a transplant, patients have a catheter (Hickman catheter) surgically implanted into the Subclavian vein in the chest. It's used for direct access to the bloodstream to give IV medications and chemo. Patients receiving high-dose chemo get mouth sores and need IV narcotics for pain control as well as IV food: TPN and lipids. As the white blood count starts to grow, the mouth sores heal, as does the whole body. Patients take an anti-rejection medication called Cyclosporine, so their bodies don't reject the donor's marrow. It runs in a continuous IV for twenty-three hours a day, thus leaving only an hour for the patient to shower and be reconnected to their medications.

5. Lymphoma is cancer of the lymphatic system. "Lymphoma occurs when lymphocytes, a type of white blood cell, grow abnormally. The body has two main types of lymphocytes that can develop into lymphomas: B-lymphocytes (B-cells) and T-lymphocytes (T-cells)." "The World Health Organization estimates that there are at least 61 types of non-Hodgkin lymphoma (NHL). Although the various types of NHL have some things in common, they differ in their appearance under the microscope, their molecular features, their growth patterns, their impact on the body and how they are treated."

   Lymphoma Research Foundation. (2012). *Lymphoma.* Retrieved May 21,2013, from http://www.lymphoma.org

6. A PET scan (positron emission topography) is a procedure that involves being injected with an IV radioactive isotope. Like a detection system, the radioactive isotope finds "hot spots," binding with cells that multiply rapidly using glucose in their growth activity. Since cancer cells are fast growing, they require a lot of energy. The purpose of the test was to identify if there were more areas of cancer, other than my groin lymph nodes. Prior to the test, a patient has his or her glucose level checked.

7. The diaphragm is a muscle below the ribcage that allows us to breathe. Involvement on both sides of the diaphragm means its spread further, hence, needs more treatment.

8. The chemo regimen called CHOP includes: C for Cytoxan (cyclophosphamide); H for hydroxydaunorubicin (doxorubicin); O for Oncovin (vincristine); and P for prednisone, which is taken orally for five days during the week chemo was given.

9. Some chemo is extremely corrosive to veins, so a port is used to give access to the Subclavian vein, one of the large veins of the blood stream. A port is a silver-dollar-sized round disc implanted into the upper chest, below the collarbone. It's placed under the skin and sticks out about an inch.

10. The pleural space is a membrane that encases the lungs. A pneumothorax is a collapse of the lung, due to air in the pleural space. (Mine was minimal, but excruciating nonetheless.)

Porth, C. (1986). *Pathophysiology: Concepts of Altered HealthStates*(Seconded.)Philadelphia,PA:J.B.Lippincott Company.

11. Prednisone is used in many forms of cancer treatment to help decrease swelling of the tumor(s). In the case of NHL, it helps kill the cancerous white blood cells.

Cancer Treatment. (2013). *Prednisone Cancer Treatment.* Retrieved on January 13, 2013, from www://prednisone.cancertreatment.net/

12. Chemotherapy is usually administered every three weeks. Chemo is targeted to kill cancer cells, but unfortunately, it also kills the fast-growing cells of the body, such as those in the gastrointestinal tract, causing nausea, thickened saliva, and sometimes mouth sores. Skin and hair follicles are also fast-growing; thus, when a patient receives certain types of chemo, he or she can also suffer from hair loss and skin dryness. Chemo is also immunosuppressive, meaning it destroys rapidly dividing cells such as white blood cells, making a person more susceptible to infection. Red blood cells, which carry the oxygen-transport protein hemoglobin as well as platelets (that help stop bleeding), are also affected, causing fatigue and making a person more susceptible to bleeding. The term "nadir" refers to the time when the blood counts reach their lowest levels during chemo, which is usually from around day seven to day fourteen. Each kind of chemo has a wide range of side effects specific to its type.

    Chemocare. (2013). *Chemotherapy.* Retrieved May 23, 2013, from http://www.chemocare.com

13. Rituxan is an IV monoclonal antibody that works to bind and destroy a specific antigen (protein), CD-20, found on the surface of B cells. It is specifically targeted to kill the non-Hodgkin lymphoma cancer cell and isn't harmful to other cells, unlike chemo. It is used in other diseases with

excessive numbers of B cells and can have side effects such as fever, body aches, hypotension, tumor lysis syndrome, or allergic reaction.

Rituxan. (2013). *Rituxan.* Retrieved May 19, 2013, from http://www.rituxan.com

14. Chemo brain is a phenomenon many cancer patients have when they receive chemotherapy. The cause is unknown, but the symptoms can include difficulty concentrating, confusion, short-term memory problems, and a feeling of mental fogginess.

Mayo Clinic.(2012). *Chemo Brain.* Retrieved on May 25, 2013, from http://www.mayoclinic.com/health/chemo-brain

15. Anticipatory nausea or vomiting is when a patient has a response to sights, smells, or sounds related to a memory of previous treatment and has an immediate response of throwing up or dry heaving.

WebMD. (2014). *Nausea and Vomiting (PDQ)*:Supportive Care-Patient Information-[NCI]-General Information. Retreived December, 23, 2014, from http://www.webmd.com/cancer/tc/nausea-and-vomiting-pdq-supportive-care---patient-information-nci-general-information

16. Cancer patients must be extra careful to take precautions from getting sick. Hand washing is a must, as well as staying away from sick contacts, especially during the time of a patient's nadir (the lowest level to which the white blood cells drop). Also, some chemotherapy can make a person more sensitive to the sun.

17. Marinol is a derivative of cannabis. It is synthetic THC, approved by the FDA, which had been found to relieve nausea and vomiting associated with chemotherapy.

    U.S. Department of Justice. Drug Enforcement Administration.(2011). *The DEA position on Marijuana.* Washington D.C: Government Printing Office. Retrieved on January 6, 2013, from http://www.justice.gov.dea/docs/marijuana_position_2011.pdf

18. Armstrong, L., Jenkins, S. *It's Not About the Bike: My journey back to life.* New York, NY. Berkley Publishing Co.

19. Some patients develop post-traumatic stress disorder while going through the trauma of cancer and treatment. This is an anxiety disorder developed in response to a severe trauma. Symptoms can include nightmares, intrusive thoughts, sleep disturbances, avoidance of the situation, and irritability.

National Cancer Institute. (2012). *Post Traumatic Stress Disorder and Cancer*. Retrieved on March 29, 2012, from www.cancer.gov/cancertopics/pdq/supportivecare/PostTraumaticstress/HealthProfessional/page1-3

20. A saline lock is an IV that is capped off without fluids going through.

21. "Adenopathy means enlargement of the lymph node." Related to a disease process.

Adenopathy. (2012). In *The Free Dictionary*. Retrieved July 2, 2012, from www.thefreedictionary.com/adenopathy

22. Chemotherapy is toxic, so it destroys red blood cells and white blood cells, taking them to dangerously low levels. Neupogen is a medication used to stimulate the growth of neutrophils, a type of white blood cell that helps the body fight infection. Common side effects are bone pain and itching or redness at the site of injection. Epogen helps increase the red blood cells (hemoglobin), thus making a patient less prone to anemia.

Neupogen. (2013). *Neupogen Side Effects*. Retrieved September 1, 2013, from www.neupogen.com

23. Because chemo is toxic it sometimes, due to the trauma it causes in the body, throws a woman into early menopause. The body can recover and reverse out of it, but that doesn't always happen.

    The Cleveland Clinic. (2013). *Menopause and Chemotherapy*. Retrieved on January 13, 2013, from http://my.clevelandclinic.org/services/chemotherapy/hic_menopause_and_chemotherapy.aspx

24. Adriamycin (doxorubicin) is a chemo drug that can be damaging to the heart (cardio toxic). Zinecard (dexrazoxane) helps protect the heart from the cardio toxic side effects.

    Chemocare. (2013). *Adriamycin and Zinecard.* Retrieved May 26, 2013, from http://www.chemocare.com

25. There are many risk factors that can lead to cancer. Working with pesticides is a risk factor for non-Hodgkin lymphoma. However, when a person is diagnosed, there is never a firm answer as to what caused it, due to how a person's body reacts to the environment, hereditary factors, and diet. There is no way to track its origin, at least in my case. Today, much more research is being done in regards to genetic factors.

Lymphoma Research Foundation. (2012). *Risk Factors.* Retrieved May 26, 2013, from http://www.lymphoma.org

26. One of the possible side effects from the chemo drug vincristine is peripheral neuropathy, damage to nerves. A patient can feel tingling, discomfort, numbness, or a pins-and-needles feeling.

Peripheral Neuropathy. (2012). In *Wikipedia.* Retrieved on January 8, 2013, from http://wikipedia.org/wiki/Peripehral_neuropathy

27. Cancer patients transitioning from treatment to survivorship sometimes deal with cancer-specific concerns. The biggest is fear of recurrence, but they can also include fear of the future, trouble sleeping, fatigue, depression, and trouble concentrating. It's important for cancer survivors to continue being monitored by the medical team for recurrence, late effects of treatment, and potential secondary malignancies. They also might have socioeconomic concerns, issues with fertility, or problems with intimate relationships, depending on how much the disease and treatment has disrupted their life. Many cancer survivors have an enhanced appreciation for life.

Committee on Cancer Survivorship: Improving Care and Quality of Life. National Cancer Policy Board. (2006). *From Cancer patient to Cancer Survivor: Lost in Transition.* Washington D.C. The National Academies Press.

28. Some patients who relapse (return of the disease) from Acute Myelogenous Leukemia (AML) may need a bone marrow transplant or stem cell transplant to increase the chances for long-term remission.

National Marrow Donor Registry. (2013). *Acute Myelogenous Leukemia.* Retrieved October 30, 2013, from http://bethematch.org/Patient/Disease_and_Treatment/About_Your_Disease/AML/Transplant_results.aspx

29. Prior to starting chemotherapy, a nurse's standard protocol is to check for a blood return (when a nurse withdraws blood from the IV line with a syringe to make sure it's in place). Patients who undergo a transplant have a Hickman catheter, or other venous access device, implanted in the chest. Tubes protrude from the chest and are used for IV and blood-drawing purposes.